Disposable Heroes

Disposable Heroes

Dan Heidt

Writers Club Press
San Jose New York Lincoln Shanghai

Writers Club Press
an imprint of iUniverse.com, Inc.

For information address:
iUniverse.com, Inc.
5220 S 16th, Ste. 200
Lincoln, NE 68512
www.iuniverse.com

Although based upon the author's experiences with NYC EMS,
this book is a work of fiction. Names, characters, places,
and incidends either are the product of the author's imagination
or are used ficttiously, and any resemblence to actual persons,
living or dead, events, or locales is entirely coincidental.

ISBN: 0-595-16602-4

Printed in the United States of America

INTRODUCTION

The silhouette of Tom taking a piss on the rear of the rig is shining under the full moon. It's my first night as a medic in Harlem. I'm riding with the senior medic and we're out of the station a whole five minutes before we get a job. As soon as we get parked by the graveyard on 155th St, the radio chimes "19–X-ray…One–Eight–Three and Wadsworth for the cardiac arrest." Tom is pissed, "19–Victor can't even pick up their own fuckin' jobs," he tells me. I don't know what's going on I'm just happy to be here. After all, I'm gonna save the world. Anyway, Tom hits the 63 responding button and tells Central we'll be extended from our area. As we travel to our job we pass four other parked units. I am baffled that no other closer unit will pick up this job, but I'll learn real fast. When we arrive, we hike our equipment up the five flights to the apartment. We find a 57-year-old asthmatic dead on the floor next to his bed. His nebulizer is still pumping out a mist of provental that didn't quite get the job done this time. Tom tells me "at least he went down fighting," as he notices about a half dozen empty tiny bottles of medication on the floor.

I'm extremely juiced and ready for battle. Tom has been here a thousand times and knows the inevitable outcome of this scenario. But I guess he wants to see if I can cut it. So he tells me to do the tube while he sets up the line. I hit the tube and started to breathe for this man. Tom hit the line and we work the arrest to no avail. Eventually we have to call medical control to pronounce death.

I'm thinking OK, what do I tell this guy's son, but I didn't have to say anything. He knew his dad wasn't going to come back, and Tom did all the talking. Telling him all that could be done was, and that he was sorry we couldn't do more. We had to leave the body with PD to move on to the next job. When we got down to the rig I felt bad that reality never really gave us a chance to do anything to bring this guy back. I was told I did a good job, but I had to calm down, cause I'm too hyper. This is something I couldn't help, and eventually caused me a lot of problems. We got back to our spot. Tom left the rig running cause he knew it was going to be one of those nights.

Before I could even get my breath back the radio called "19–X-ray…One–Six–Nine and Haven for the unconscious." Tom was pissed again "right around the corner from the fucking hospital" he tells me, "but at least it's a street job." When we get there it turns out to be a kid about 20, drunk off his ass, laying in a puddle of green lumpy puke. I really want to make my partner happy, so I tell him I'll work this one, no problem. So we get him on the stretcher, and in the rig. Since he has nice young, large veins, the line goes in easier than sex. Narcan, dextrose and thiamin do nothing for him, so we transport him to the ER. After the job is done, we find out in the ER that this is a third year med student. Tom is laughing as we leave and he tells me "Can you believe that asshole is going to be a doctor?" I think I can cause I know where I come from, and it's a lot worse than what I just saw.

So we get in the rig. We don't even leave the hospital and we get a job. "19–X-ray…One–Two–Two and Park for the unconscious." "Great," he tells me, "This is 17 Willie's job and we're more than 80 blocks away." When we get there we find some 60 pound crack-head that's telling Tom to get the fuck away from him. "I didn't call no fuckin' ambulance and I ain't sick." Tom is telling me this is a good job, cause he can walk and we can take him to Met (a hospital on Nine–Six and Two). But he don't want to go anywhere with us, so we make him a 93 (patient refused all care) and then we move on. We can't seem to get back to our own area. We're heading up St. Nicholas Avenue, when we get another job. "19–X-ray…One–Four–Five and Lenox for the sick." Well let me tell you, I thought my partner was going to have a stroke. "A sick job is BLS not ALS, where the hell are all the BLS units?" When we got to the scene, we found an emaciated 50-year-old man in a roach infested apartment, with no furniture. Tom talks to him and we find out this guy's a Vietnam veteran, we also find out he hasn't eaten in three days and he doesn't want to go to the hospital either. Tom talks to him about 10 minutes, and then to my surprise he gives the guy $10 and asks him to buy some food in the morning. I was very surprised he did this. But I would end up gaining an incredible amount of respect for Tom, by the end of the night. It turns out that Tom too is a Vietnam veteran and earned a Purple Heart among his many commendations for being wounded in combat. It seems Tom left half his intestines in some rice paddy ten thousand miles away, while I was in kindergarten. By the time I even had ball hair, Tom had been doing this job more than ten years. I decided I was going to do everything I could to make his job easier. But I had a real hard time, cause I was way too hyper and emotional. I think it took a year and a half before Tom would even acknowledge me as a real medic.

So were not even through my first night and I had already done more than my entire career in the privates, where I had been doing the renal roundup for the past three years. We finally got a chance to breathe, when we heard the radio go again. This time it was 18 Young. "One–Three–Eight and Powell for the cardiac arrest." It turns out that night Tom's partner Rich was on 18 Young, working with Jason. Jason came out of the Academy with me, and Rich and Tom had to be split up cause they couldn't put two newjacks out alone. That's why Tom was pissed most of the night. Anyway we cruise by their job. I guess so Tom could make sure his partner was all right. Rich, who was also a senior medic, is letting Jason do a lot of work. Their arrest is not going so well. There's a lot of puke on the floor and the family's hysterical. Their patient doesn't come back either.

After the job I was talking with Jason. I was surprised how upset he was. He told me his night wasn't going so well and he was thinking about quitting, cause he wasn't getting it. I told him my night sucked too, but we would be all right. I also told him I thought my partner hated me. I said that some day we would work together, we would make a difference, we would kick-ass and do a lot more than just play with mannequins, like we did at the Academy. Talk about being disillusioned, I think about that night now and say to myself, I would have kicked my ass too. So the night moved on and I watched the sun finally come. I thought I was going to finish up soon. Sorry there goes the radio again. I really grew to hate that voice that I would never see. "19–X-ray…One–Five–Eight and Amsterdam for the jumper down." Great, I'm really juiced now. Tom just wants to go home. We pull up the block, next to an abandoned building, and it turns out that this job is referred to as crack-head gets a flying lesson. This guy had been burning all night, when he finally became too much of a pain in the ass for his party buddies. He got himself thrown out of the building the quick way—out the third floor window. So he's lying in a big pile of garbage, he got a broken wrist and lots of abrasions. But he's not really broken up too bad. His blood pressure is low, but probably a result of his physical long-term condition, than the fall. I work en route to the hospital, after this guy is immobilized on the board. I drop a 14 gauge IV in his good arm, splint the broken one, and arrive at Harlem hospital as I'm tying the splint. We get our paper work finished, and I could tell Tom had a long night with me, so I'm keeping my mouth shut. We get in the station, sign our drugs back in, and our lieutenant breaks the good news to Tom. Jeff banged in, Sorry but I've got to mandate you. I think Tom expected this, but he was still pissed. I couldn't imagine making a person stay a minimum of six more hours after a night like that, but I think the lieutenant enjoyed it. I found out that we would get mandated 2-3 times a week, and that this night wasn't even considered busy. Holy Shit. Anyway, I went home, Tom stayed. Two hours of traffic, and a $7 toll later, I was home. I slept like the dead we pronounced earlier and then went back to start the whole endless process again.

CHAPTER 1

I wasn't born super medic; I'm probably still not. But at least I think I am. So that's OK. I started out a low-level reefer dealer in Bensonhurst. My father was a real scumbag, a bully. I could never do anything right. Can you imagine getting 3 A's and 2 B's on a report card, and getting abused and grounded for this? I was always a quitter, a loser, and an embarrassment. The whole world was right, I was always wrong. Guilty until proven guilty. The guy would go out of his way to show he didn't have any favoritism towards his own family. When I finally left, I didn't realize how fucked up things were until I was finally away from him. So how does a sixteen-year-old survive? I made friends with some gangsters and started to sell weed. I did this for a long time. Justifying it by telling myself, I pay my bills. I'm not on welfare. I don't hold my hand out to anyone. I was very unhappy. Inevitably at 28, I got busted with 9 guns and 75 pounds of weed. I found myself unskilled with no practical experience, and a six-month-old daughter. I was extremely depressed and Prozac was not working. Someone I respected very much told me that I was becoming like a horse that's been whipped too much. Once the horse's spirit is broken it never comes back, he said. You're a good guy there's a lot you can do. I was given a 1/2 ounce of gongie, and told go roll a few fat ones. Sit in a place of peace and figure out what you can do. I thought this was good advice and I was happy to be able to get high again. But I didn't know where to start. My buddy later told me to get the yellow pages. Everything in there is legal and makes someone money. So I rolled 5 of the fattest bones I ever smoked. I took my radio and my Doors tapes. I went to the beach, put on the Soft Parade, and started to go through the Yellow Pages to find my destiny. I figured I would make a list of things I could do. I finally narrowed this list to Veterinarian or Paramedic. I didn't have time or money to go to Veterinary school, but I knew I could become an EMT relatively quickly and produce a paycheck. I was still facing charges and the very real possibility of going upstate for a very long time. Anyway I decided I would go on an absolute, fight for my life, will not be denied mission. A job with honor, something my kids could be proud of. Something I didn't have to hide. I wasn't even sure I would be allowed to sit for the state test, but what the fuck did I have to lose?

I was still very depressed; my grandfather had recently been killed by a cop car and a stolen car that crashed into him at a red light. My rottweiler got hip displasia, and had to be put to sleep. I went from making $1500 a week, clear tax-free to working under the steaming July sun at a gas station for $4 an hour off the books. I took my EMT class and half way through, needed surgery on my knee. If I had more than 3 absences I would be out. I had to borrow the money for this class from my brother, who to this day has never even asked for this money back. There was no tomorrow for me, I had to pass this course. So I hobbled through the last half, and by some miracle of God, I was able to sit for the state test, which I got an 85 on. I then received 5 years probation from the judge, which was another miracle and I got a job as an EMT. I thought that everyone who did this job had a good heart and was an honorable person. Man, was I wrong. I was a depressed rookie. People cut the line to kick me when I was down. People, who six months ago, I wouldn't have pissed on if they were on fire, were dumping all their own shit on this easy mark of a know-nothing rookie.

It took me about a week to realize this job wasn't on the level, but I was working (my first real job). I remember waking up at 5 in the morning to take people to and from dialysis for ten hours a day. I thought I was going to save lives, but I was nothing more than a well-lit taxicab.

I stuck with it and got myself into medic school. I had no clue what I was getting into. I had to work weekend doubles 7 to 11 on Saturdays, 10 to 2 on Sundays, and then 5 am to 1 on Tuesdays to get my 40 hours. I traveled through rush-hours traffic Monday through Friday to be in the classroom from 6 to 10, and did 1,060 hours of unpaid clinical rotations on overnights. I was burnt before I even started being a medic, but I worked really hard. I knew little to nothing and was very opinionated and at times very judgmental. I quickly gained the negative attention of my senior instructor who became determined to fail me out of this class.

Fortunately for myself, other people were able to see the real me. I made allies with a lot of people who had credibility. People who would also cross my path in a positive way at the Academy and in Harlem. I felt that my soul had a big hole in it and that I was covered with scar tissue. I knew if I could just remove the blackness that society and my father inflicted on me that I could be a good guy, a good father and a good medic. This struggle continues even today. Getting through medic school was the hardest thing I ever did in my life.

My second daughter was born right at the beginning of this class. So having a newborn didn't exactly help with the stress of probation, the job, and medic school. I still don't know how I got through. Maybe there is an EMS God.

I got a job as a medic in Staten Island as soon as I graduated. I wasn't doing any meaningful work, but now at least I was making $16.50 an hour. I couldn't shake depression and quickly found others taking advantage of this. My second daughter was extremely difficult to take care of. I had to work nights so my wife could work days. I still didn't know my kid had autism. I found this out at 18 months of age after she had a seizure and had to be transported to the ER. Anyway fate intervened again and I got a call from the EMS academy. I could start there in the next medic class upgrade, if I was available. This was a good break, because I was about to be fired like a cannon from my present job.

I got to the Academy and I actually had the audacity to think I was a medic already. After all, I had the patch, right? I was quickly slapped down and encouraged to quit. "Fuck you," I thought, "no one here is any better than me." But this was hollow thinking, and I really needed to prove that to myself.

At the Academy is where I met Jason, who I never realized would be my favorite partner. He was genuinely nice to me without expecting to gain anything, and was one of the people who got me through. I turned a lot of people off, but I also continued to gain allies with the people I respected. When I finally graduated from the EMS Academy, Jason and I were assigned to Manhattan along with two other guys Phil and Shaffee. Both of whom are also genuinely good guys and excellent medics.

I volunteered to go to Station 18 (Harlem). There were two openings there and two openings at station 15 (Metropolitan). Jason got assigned Harlem, based on having the lowest social security number, the rest is history.

In Harlem is where I made my stand with the best partner a man could ask for. A partner you could trust and rely on. Only people in EMS know how few real partners you get in this industry. In Jason I had a partner I could go into battle with, any night, any weather, any job, any disease, anywhere, unconditionally, no questions asked. I could be myself. We could work like animals and truly be productive. A lot of the best jobs we ever did I wouldn't have been able to pull off with any other partner. I actually got into a parking lot fistfight, because I wouldn't let someone refer to him as puppy medic. When we were on 16–Victor, I felt like we were kings of the city and I will go into this in great detail in future chapters.

CHAPTER 2

So when I got to the station for my second night, I found out the hard way just how under the microscope I was. My reputation had preceded me to the station, and it was not going to be easy to gain respect or be accepted. Apparently when you're a good guy nobody notices. But people who talk better than they produce always find a way to get the focus off of themselves and onto the newjack.

There hadn't been new medics in Harlem for three years so everyone there had light years of experience on me both politicking and with patient care. Tom told me in order to be successful in EMS you needed to be anonymous. But I had already blown that up when I was at the Academy riding rotations in the South Bronx.

We encountered a real skell unit 22–Frank (BLS). What went down was really fucked-up. We get a sick job, some 200 pound plus solid young woman with abdominal pain. She's on the 6th floor and the elevator is broken (big surprise). Anyway this unit backs us up cause they want to check out the new crop of rookies. I assess the patient with my partner, Derrick and under the watchful eyes of our preceptor we decide it's in our best interest to carry her. While I'm setting up he stair chair this asshole, Cherise tells the woman "come on the elevator is broken, not your legs." So when I told her we've gotta carry this patient, she laughs at me and tells me "little boy you need to come to the Bronx and learn the way things are done." Well that pushed my button good. I told her "in the real world, I would 84 this patient to a BLS unit." But since I cared about people she could take a hike and was 87'd (an 84 is no need for medics; 87 is you're not needed).

So me and Derrick are carrying this woman, and all the way down this BLS bitch is saying "good thing you ate your Wheaties," and "come on your not carrying her right." While not lifting a finger to help us. When we got down to the rig, I stepped out and before Two–Two–Frank left, I told Cherise she was a fucking skell and if I came to the Bronx I would be her worst nightmare. Anyway I had a real attitude problem now. So when I'm in the back of the rig with my patient and her sister, I found out they both liked me, and felt really good that me and Derrick did the right thing. Outside the ER, my patient's sister came and gave me a matchbook with her number and told me to call her sometime. I didn't think I would, but something told me to keep the number, and I'm lucky I did.

So I'm outside the ER at St. Barnabus and these two EMT's come up to me and tell me you really know how to make friends don't you. You really pissed off Cherise good. I responded in vintage Dan form "Fuck that stupid bitch, I can't wait to get home so I can think about her when I jerk-off." Well of course the wrong person heard this, and next thing you know the whole fucking Bronx is talking about this newjack asshole rookie, and they all think I'm going to be an easy mark. So Cherise files this EEO against me. Some bureaucratic smoke screen bullshit to cover up her own incompetent patient care.

Anyway, I'm on the verge of getting kicked out of the Academy for doing the right thing, and having a mouth that would make Ralph Kramden look like a mime. So I'm feeling real shitty and I'm thinking where can I look for a new job. I called the girl who gave her number to me. I told her I'm in a lot of trouble over this bullshit, and I'm probably going to lose my job before I even start.

Well it turns out this woman is a cop in the Four–Four Precinct. She knew Cherise and her partner were scumbags. She wrote a letter to the Academy telling them how they treated her sister like shit on their shoes, and that me and Derrick were the greatest things since the invention of hot chocolate. This saved my ass but I was marked for doom. When I got to

Harlem, everyone already knew about this incident and it took a long time to live down.

I worked with Rich my second night, while Jason worked with Tom. I immediately liked Rich, we really thought alike on a lot of issues. I knew he would give me a chance and judge me on my virtues, not the hearsay of nauseating malcontents that just talk so much shit while producing nothing. Besides Rich thought this story was hysterical. He told me I should of mooned her and told her to kiss my brown eye.

So my first job with Rich is some idiot with the flu. "18–Young One–Four–Four and Douglas for the 24 year old with difficulty breathing." We get there and Rich asks this guy what changed in the last 4 days that you gotta have an ambulance now. The guy just looks at him and says "Que. No Ingles," as he shows us a pot of puke. Rich tells him OK lets go. It seems our boy understands English just fine, even if he makes like he can't speak it. We get him to the rig, he's warm, BP of 120/80 heart rate of 84 and coughing all over the fucking place. Rich tells me nothing like a real emergency, huh, as he hands me the Medicaid card. He puts a non-rebreather on him, and tells me this is for our own protection. Who knows, maybe its tuberculosis he says. We take the guy to Columbia Presbyterian and the nurse scribbles on the ACR and tells me let him sit in the waiting area. So Hector starts holding his chest like he's dying, but know one is buying it. He's gonna sit till sunrise, bet on it.

Our second job was a good one. A straight up 78-year-old cardiac arrest. This woman is still warm and definitely workable. Rich started CPR, while I set up the tube. No resistance, no puke, easy visualization of the vocal cords. I thought is looked like a white vagina as I passed the tube through and started to breathe for her. Rich took over the tube and also let me do the line. This was great, I was doing all the work and I was getting it right. She was flat-line the whole way, nothing changed. I wound up dumping 6 epi's and 3 atropines in her. I ran AMS too. I was excited, but I felt fucked-up afterwards cause I thought someone died and I was thinking what a great job it was.

Rich liked me, I know he did and he enjoyed teaching. I was going to work hard for him. The night went fast. In the morning when Rich was going to get mandated, I told the lieutenant I would stay instead. I wound up working 6 hours overtime and didn't get home till 3:30 in the afternoon. I still had to deal with my kids who didn't want to understand overtime, and be back at midnight. But at least today, I was happy.

When I went back to work, the first person I saw was Jason. He told me that Rich was saying good things about me, and didn't mind working with me. He also told me I would be working with Tom again tonight, and he would be working with Rich. I was glad I made a good impression with Rich, and I knew I was going to be a good boy tonight with Tom. This was a Friday night, usually the busiest night of the week. I was ready to rock, but Tom was tired. He wanted a slow night, but he knew there was no such thing. We signed our drugs and checked out the rig. We weren't even done checking our shit out when it came—"19–X-ray, are you in service yet," the radio blared. Tom answered not at this time. But Central didn't give a shit. "19–X-ray, you have an assignment. One–Seventeen and St. Nick for the confirmed shot." "Fuck," Tom yelled at the drug box. "Come on, let's go," he told me. We got rolling and the sirens screamed. I thought my head was going to pop. I was so juiced…I was electric. Anyway, when we get to the scene, it's chaos. People are all around, cops everywhere. This guy is up against the wall shot four times, close range, in the face and head. His brains are on the wall, and his head looks like an isosceles triangle. This guy is toast. We're not going to work, and Tom is relaxed. I'm pacing like a caged tiger. It's a crime scene. "Don't touch nothing," I'm told. "Don't even fuckin' breathe near him." We're out of service doing paper work for a while. No carry down, no puke, no aggravation, just bullshit with the detectives for a while. Tom likes this, and all the cops know him. It's a social gathering now. The veteran medics and the cops are numb to this. They block it out easy. I will learn how to do this too, and I'll become quite good at it. But for now, all I'm seeing is the army-green brain matter splattered on a blue wall, with a puddle of thick crimson blood flowing down the sidewalk and into the gutter. I'm thinking, "wow this is fucked-up," but you know what, it ain't shit. Its all been done before and its still being done after I'm gone. Besides the night is still young and there's more to come. I just don't realize how much. But at least I feel devirgined now.

So, we've been out of service about 45 minutes, when our patrol supervisor comes to the scene to break our balls to go back in service. This lieutenant is a big fat female, and I didn't need Tom to explain to me that her greatest talent was lifting the fork off the plate. Anyway we're in the St. Luke's area now and as soon as we go available, we get a job—Is there a pattern emerging yet? "19–X-ray, One–Eleven and B'way for the dif breather on the street." I ask Tom, "are they fuckin' kidding?" This guy is standing on the corner of the hospital. Not only that 16–Willy whose job it should have been, is parked one short block away holding their damn signal. So now I knew why they were referred to as 16–Worthless around the station. A title this unit would continually reinforce on all three tours.

So we get to the corner, and this fucking guy is standing there smoking a cigar, telling us he's got asthma. So I tell him "Why the fuck don't you just walk into the hospital" (What a concept huh). So it turns out this guy is a regular. I would wind up doing him about 20 times over the next year. His game was to get you to give him a provental nebulizer treatment, then refuse transport (RMA). The treatment would then open up his breathing passages and then he would go smoke crack. Your taxes at work I thought. This fuckin guy is living in a city shelter, on welfare his whole life, and using food stamps to trade for crack at 25 cents on a dollar. (Never underestimate the importance of taking a good history). After a while I didn't mind this guy, cause he always took us out of service for about forty minutes, and we would end up on 110 and B'way. This was the only place to get decent food in the middle of the night. So I decide to treat myself to an onion bagel with lox and cream cheese, and a nice hot coffee. I really got to like this and would become a regular at the bagel spot there. Tom would get tea, and at 60 cents a cup, I could be a sport.

Our night continues, and I was already starting to see how this job could really fuck you up. I mean the job was bad enough, but then you had all these people who were supposed to be on your team constantly fucking you. Especially useless lieutenants and captains who had to justify their existence by producing large quantities of paperwork. I was really happy to be a poor bureaucrat and politician. But I learned fast this was going to fuck me, but I really didn't care. I don't want to give the impression that I thought all the lieutenants were assholes. A lot are, and were very cool. And a few really looked out for us. But the ones that were out to make your life miserable had a master's degree and a natural ability to do it.

I actually got to finish my bagel before the next one came over. "19–X-ray…One–Four–Nine and Riverside Drive for the unconscious." So I'm reading the text of the KDT (the vehicles onboard computer). It's pretty funny. It states 28-year female caller says she's unconscious. Now, I'm getting pissed. Tom tells me "get used to it." I'm saying "what a great trick, you're unconscious, but you can call and use the telephone." So we get to the building along with PD at the same time. A lot of kids are hanging out in the lobby. The smell of crack is almost as strong as Clorox bleach. They don't even notice us or the cops. Or at least they don't seem to. We get to an elevator that actually works, and we travel up to the fifth floor. In the elevator the smell of old piss alleviates the smell of crack. When we get to the apartment, the smell of garbage, older than me, wipes out the smell of the piss. I ask this woman "who's unconscious?" And she tells me "I was unconscious you stupid motherfucker," as she's crying "I gotta get this tooth pulled—take me to Harlem hospital." Well now at least the smell of her breath has wiped out the smell of garbage. We take her to our taxi and Tom explains that she has to go to CPMC, cause that's the closest hospital. He tells her if she wants to go to Harlem, she has to take a cab, not an ambulance.

Well she bitches all the way to Columbia. Calls me a stupid mother-fucker for about the thirty-fifth time, and doesn't even go into the emergency room. Instead, she walks over to a pay phone on the corner of One–Six–Eight and B'way, dials 911 and tells the operator she can't breath. So guess what. A minute and a half later the radio summons us—"19–X-ray...One-Six-Eight and B'way for the dif breather on the street." This puts me over the top tonight. I'm already on only two hours sleep as it is. I tell her, "come on, get the hell back in the rig, let's go." In the rig she's still telling me I'm a stupid mother-fucker. And I snapped back, "I'm a stupid mother-fucker, you're right, cause I'm here with you now." She tells me, "you shoulda just took me to Harlem in the first place, cause they got a dentist all night." Well, what the fuck do I know? It's only my third night here, I thought. This bitch has been juicing the system the past 25 years. So we get her to the hospital. I get to do double paper work, and Lieutenant Lardass is breaking our balls to get back in service before the ink is even dry on my ACR's. Tom tells me, "welcome to Station 18."

CHAPTER 3

So a few days have passed. I'm getting lots of overtime. I'm starving for acceptance, but I'm obviously going about it the wrong way. I'm working with Rich again tonight, and I'm having a decent night. He's showing me the sights of Washington Heights, and I didn't realize there really was a lot of history there. He shows me where Malcolm X was shot, and where George Washington's headquarters was. He lets me know that he remembers the night Malcolm X was shot. I said "I knew you were older than dirt, but just don't tell me your were doing jobs when George Washington was here." This made him laugh and it got my mind off the tough time I had been having.

So, it's about 3:30 in the morning, and were watching this woman pushing a baby carriage, and pulling two other kids about 2 and 4 along with her. I couldn't imagine where they were going, but I realized it was none of my business. Besides this was a very common sight.

We got a job in the subway. It came over as an altered mental status. This is EMS language for go get the fucking lunatic. Rich explained to me en route how in this job you needed to be part paramedic, part cop, part social worker, part mommy, part daddy, and of course, part garbage man. We got down in the tunnels, and it didn't take long to find this guy walking up and down the platform screaming profanities with his dick hanging out.

Obviously this person did not want to see us, or the cops. But I guess he thought his behavior was OK. Anyway, with the help of PD, we wrapped him up in a thick black wool blanket, and tied him into the stair chair. What I didn't realize was that this upstanding citizen should have also been gagged, cause he was spitting on me the whole way up the stairs. When we got him up to the rig, he decided this would be a good time to piss himself. Anyway we took him to K-Building, and although I had to clean up all this nonsense, at least we were out of service BBP (Blood Borne Pathogens). We get back in service, we do a couple more uneventful taxi type jobs, and it's real late. The sun is probably going to be up in about a half-hour, and we get a call as I started to nod out. "18–Young…One–Five–Eight and Amsterdam, for the unconscious." We're thinking it's probably a bullshit intox job, and if we're lucky our unconscious patient will be able to walk to the bus. So it turns out this guy is laying in the street, with a Frankenstein-like crack across his forehead. This moron tried to rob the diner with a broken bottle, so the guy behind the counter came around and hit him in the head with a ballpeen hammer. They then dragged him out into the street and waited for a concerned citizen to call 911.

I guess about 20 people stepped over him, before someone decided he had to be removed. So when we get there, this guy is all postured and has agonal respirations. He's completely clamped up, and his BP is 240 over 130. This is a real job. We get him on the board and collared. Rich tells me bag him on the fly, if you can get him intubated, do it. I didn't need to be told this. Besides these are the jobs a gung-ho rookie lives for. I was able to get an oral airway in and I hyperventilated him. There would be no IV; we were only a minute and a half from CPMC.

I put my legs under the stretcher and sat on the floor. I had an 8.0 ET tube set up, and used a MAC 3 laryngoscope blade. I had a literal 180-degree view of his vocal cords, as I slid the blade in and took the airway out. I got the tube in one try (it was all I was gonna get). We were at the hospital before I even had the tube secured. Before we took him out of the rig, Rich confirmed my tube was good. This earned a lot of credibility with him. I secured the tube and continued to breathe for the patient. We got into the ER, and realized our boy was going to live to rob another diner. Assuming his brain injury did not leave him impersonating a potted plant for the next 30 years.

I felt really good about being able to pull off this job, and thought is was a good night's work. But the real job came about an hour later, just as we were about to take the unit in for the tour change. We're sitting in the rig, Rich treated me to a coffee and bagel. I'm still online from our last job, when the dispatcher decided to clear her board. We listened to a rapid-fire succession of jobs go over the air. Rich knew we were going to get banged, and he was bitching how all these dispatchers are a bunch of donut-eating, 300-pound sadist. "Fuck a unit, get a Twinkie," he said. "These fucking guys have no accountability, just clear the board." "Doesn't matter if you take medic units out of service for bullshit." "If you hold your signal you get fucked. But these assholes will take you out of service four hours a night with bullshit jobs." "The goddam system just fucking proliferates itself." Sure as a sunrise, there it came. "18–Young…One–Eight–Five and Broadway for the sick." Motherfucker, not only was this a late job, but it was a BLS late job, way out of our area. Needless to say we were both extremely torched. So we get there thinking its bullshit. The KDT is saying 71-year-old Spanish speaking female states she's sick. Of course, she's in an apartment on the forth floor. No elevator, which is OK, cause it would probably be filled up with piss, even if it was there.

We get to a very clean well-kept apartment, as this little old lady comes to the door. She's alone in the apartment, and she can't speak any English. We immediately knew this was more than a sick job. This lady was a light shade of gray. She was cold, and diaphoretic. We sat her on the bed and Rich knew by the sound of her very labored wet breathing, that she was in pulmonary edema. I was getting a blood pressure, while Rich was putting oxygen on her. He went to get the monitor. I knew her BP was over 200, and I told him this. As he put the stickies on her chest, she dropped right in front of us. He pulled her onto the floor supine and started CPR. The patient was flat-line except for the wide complexes

Rich's CPR generated. I came around him and dropped a 7.5 tube in her. We hadn't even set a line up yet when Rich checked her for a pulse and noticed we had a sinus tach rhythm. She came back so good we had to tape her hands together to keep her from tearing the tube out. Rich quickly put an 18-gauge IV in her right forearm, gave her lasix, and we proceeded to hike her down the four flights of stairs. Stopping on every landing to ventilate her. We got onto the rig, and asked dispatch to notify CPMC that we were coming in with a resuscitation, post arrest vitals, rate of 120, BP 100 over 70, respirations assisted. We were in the ER in about 4 minutes. The whole job took less than 30 minutes 63 to 81 (en route till we got to the hospital). When we were leaving to go home, this lady's grandson was coming in.

Someone must have pointed us out to him, cause he rushed over to us shaking our hands and telling us in broken English we were heroes. I felt so good my stomach was tingling, and I was sweating so much it looked like someone dumped a bucket of ice water on me. I felt better than Michael Jordan hitting a three-pointer with no time left that won a playoff game. I had temporarily even forgotten the previous job. I only remembered when the triage nurse came over and told me "Boy you guys had a great night." I got home that morning and I couldn't wait to tell my wife and daughter what we had done. The ride home took like no time. I floated in my door and was so electrified I couldn't sleep all day. I couldn't wait to get back to work that night. I didn't care what unit I was working and who I was working with. But I knew Rich would always be one of my favorite partners.

CHAPTER 4

So I'm struggling on the plantation. I'm starting to realize in this system, I'm not Dan Heidt, I'm robotic ambulance driver number 3908. Work till you drop, then be replaced by another 3908.

On this particular night I was supposed to work with Brendan. Brendan had a big time rep at the station. I immediately thought of him as the Clint Eastwood of medics. He was tough and stocky. He carried a lot of equipment on his belt and had been known to take a lot of dynamite pictures. He had made it abundantly clear that he didn't care much for me. I know he thought he was getting fucked by having to work with me. I had never been with Brendan before and I couldn't understand what I had done to him. I must admit that I was kind of intimidated by him, which doesn't happen much to me. But after all, I was still a new-jack rookie. Brendan is a real pit bull, but you know what, I'm a pit bull too and someday we will work together, and we won't allow ourselves to fuck up in front of each other.

I now think of Brendan as another of my favorite partners. Who probably still doesn't realize how high of a regard I hold him in. I didn't know what a kick ass partner I had till we didn't work together anymore. Before we even signed out our drugs fate intervened. So what happened, how come we didn't work together that night? Well, Tom was supposed to work with Robin. She's a skinny little, scrawny, four-eyed, man-hating dyke and a poor medic on top of that. (Did I mention that I'm very opinionated?) Anyway, this douche bag gets on Tom's unit, and sits behind the steering wheel. She tells him to check out the equipment, cause it's her night to drive and she's a medic just like him. Well you know what, even I was never that dumb!

Tom didn't say a word. He just went to the back of the rig. He took her bags off the bus, and just fuckin' flung them onto Lenox Avenue. Then, he went around, opened the driver side door and told her "get the fuck off my unit." He went inside and told Lieutenant Lardass, he would not work with this idiot, and he was going home sick. Well, guess who got to work with Robin that night? Tom went into service with Brendan on 19–X-ray. I had one of the longest nights of my career with Robin on 18 Young.

So we get in service, and it takes about 5 minutes before she's telling me I just better do what I'm told, and that she's the senior medic on the rig tonight. I'm trying to be a conformist so I'm just thinking about seeing my daughters in the morning, and not about how miserable I'm going to be tonight.

Our first job is a 300-pound, 55-year-old man, who's having chest pain. He's legit, and has a history of unstable angina. Robin blows the line in his arm, and he has no real visible veins. His BP is 140 over 90, and I want to give him a nitro, after putting oxygen on him. But Robin's got to have a line, before we can give him the nitro. Oh, by the way, did I mention that we're on a hundred and thirty-fifth and Powell, thirty seconds away from Harlem hospital. Apparently this doesn't matter to her. This patient is fully alert and anxious. I want to transport. So what happens next? She decides to try a line in his neck. I had never encountered anyone like this before. I mean, am I wrong, cause I wanted to give him the O2 and nitro, then take him around the corner? Well, of course, Dr. Robin blows his external jugular. I'm dying of embarrassment. And on top of all this, she walks him out to the rig, cause she couldn't even carry one of this guy's arms, let alone his body.

Our second job is a 21-year-old female asthmatic. She's real tight and not moving any air. We give her a nebulizer treatment, and it's doing nothing. I want to get the order for epi, but Dr. Robin notices this woman is throwing about 6 PVC's a minute, and she wants to give this patient lidocane. I suggested the PVC's were probably due to hypoxia, and we should treat the patients presenting problem. You know, the one where she can't breathe. So, we don't give epi or lidocane, we just transport, and I'm thinking, damn, I hope I don't have to explain any of this to the captain. We get a bit of a break before we're sent to our next job. It's a 60-year-old unconscious female. After we're let into the apartment, I see the drugs on the bureau, and that one of the drugs she takes is glyburide, but of course, Dr. Robin thinks this woman is stroked out. She tells me, "you can't do nothing for a stroke except transport." But you know what, I may be a rookie, but I'm not a dick. Enough is enough. I tell her I have an AMS protocol to run.

She's rushing me to do the line, hanging over my shoulder like a harpy. I hit the line and start to push the dextrose through, our patient starts to come around. I give her an oral glucose. I tell her I know its tastes terrible, but please eat this. Then I asked Robin if she thought it was a hemorrhagic or thrombolytic stroke, and I'm wondering how much more of this I can take. So we go park by the triangle on St. Nick and One–three–six, now it's like 3:00 in the morning. The radio overseer summons us—"18–Young…One–Four–Six and Douglas for the dif breather." I'm already wiped out, and when we get to the scene, we've got another 300-pounder. He's pale, cool, and diaphoretic, he has a cardiac history, and he took his own nitro prior to our arrival, with no relief. Well guess what, Robin expects this guy to start doing calisthenics, to make sure he's not having muscular skeletal pain. I asked her if she was out of her fucking mind, right in front of the patient.

After we finally get out of the ER, I tell Lieutenant Lardass I won't baby-sit this incompetent idiot anymore. So now, I'm a problem. I'm told to finish the tour and keep my mouth shut. I go back into service, and thank God, the night will soon be done.

Our last job is a textbook pulmonary edema. When we walk in, the firemen are doing a blood pressure, and the woman is on oxygen. Robin asks the fireman, what he thinks is wrong with this patient. He tells her he doesn't know. So she starts going off on him, and tells him how if they're going to work with us, they got to know what they're doing.

Well this woman is bad off. I get a line, we've given three nitros, and 80 mg of lasix. I get on the phone with medical control and get an order for morphine. Nothing is really helping, and this patient is lethargic, gray and full. I decide she needed to be intubated, and I banged the tube quickly and efficiently. Robin looks at the monitor, which is flat-line, and she tells me "the patient is in arrest, begin CPR."

I nearly shit myself, thinking I just killed her. I checked for a carotid pulse, and its there—strong, about 120. I tell Robin, "I got a pulse." She gives me a death stare and says, "begin CPR." I look at the monitor, which is still flat-line, and feel the pulse. I realize that the cable is not plugged into the monitor. I inserted the cable into the monitor, and it immediately showed sinus tach. I looked back at Robin, and said sarcastically "can I have my save bar now." I then found myself apologizing to the firemen. I had to tell them how embarrassed I was to be with her. I told them "I've got no seniority and no one else back at the station will work with her." The firemen said they felt for me, and then helped us carry the lady down to the rig so she could be transported.

We finished our tour uneventfully, and as I was leaving the parking lot, I asked the EMS god to please never lift his leg on me like that again.

CHAPTER 5

I've been on the overnight tour for a while now. I've had a lot of good jobs, and I'm thinking I'm starting to get better at this. But, as it turns out the station is short of personnel on the day tours. I get called into the Captain's office, and he tells me I have got to get moved on to days for a while to cover the vacancies. This is really difficult for me, because it means I have to commute from Staten Island to Harlem, and back, in both rush hours. This trip takes over two hours each way on days, and it sucks. I get assigned to ride 18–Young, 8 to 4, with Neil and Sarge.

They're third partner will be out a few months, cause she's having a baby. Anyway, I'm meeting a lot of good people on the day tour. And there are some more of the best medics in the world working these units.

Neil and Sarge, are both excellent medics, and good guys. But at this point in my career there is still no way I'll be able to fill Debbie's shoes. They realize this, and they're both patient with me. I really like working with Neil. I'm seeing that he is highly intelligent and greatly skilled. Both of these guys cut me loose, and this enables me to get lots of experience. One day, while working with Neil, we got four arrests in a row. The first one was a pisser. It was a Saturday morning, and we got hit right out of the box. "18–Young" the radio summons, Neil answers "Young—go." "One–Three–Two and Five, for the cardiac arrest." We tell Central we're responding, and we get to an apartment that's an obvious crack den. We're led into a room that has nothing but a bar, a stereo, and a couch. On the couch is this guy, who's about 45-years-old. He's cold and he's stiff. Neil asks the person who let us in, "how long has he been like this?" The guy responds, "well, you know, we don't exactly know. We was having a party, you know, and old Harvey there, he's a diabetic, so you know, when we gots to getting down, we just figured he had a couple of drinks and nodded off." Well what little professionalism I had was very difficult to keep. I didn't want to laugh, but I really did need to leave the room for a minute. Neil told the guy, he was sorry, but there was nothing we could do for Harvey. We left the body with PD, and went to get coffee.

So now, we're down by the St. Luke's area. The radio calls, "18–Young…One–Two–Five and Amsterdam for the cardiac arrest." This job is all the way up on the eighteenth floor of the projects. A lady had tried to call her mother, like she did every morning. Only this time no one would answer the phone. She assumed her elderly mother was dead, and called 911 from her location. She told the dispatcher she thought her mother might have died. So we get up to the apartment, no one answers the door. We get ESU to come, and they knock the door in, so we can enter. We immediately see an elderly lady walking in circles, mumbling in the living room. I'm thinking she's got Alzheimer's or something, but at least it's not an arrest. Neil is trying to communicate with her to no avail. He asks me to check the medicine cabinet, so we can find out what meds she's on. This turns out to be the ultimate role reversal. Before I open the bathroom door, I notice a real foul odor coming out. I look in and there's the home attendant dead on the bowl. Her pants and underwear are down to her ankles, and although she was a black lady, her whole body was completely white, except for her head and ass, which were a deep shade of purple. I came back around and told Neil, "uh, guess what," we got an 83 in here. So this is how our day is starting. Two jobs, two DOA's, no transports. OK, so we get down to the rig, we park on One–Three–Six and St. Nick. Neil starts to read the newspaper and I step off the rig to have a cigarette. I don't even get two drags down, when the radio goes again. "18–Young…One–Six–Three and Edgecombe, for the cardiac arrest." "Young—show me 63," Neil tells dispatch. When we get in, it's a 58-year-old man, laying next to his bed in a puddle of yellow, biley, smelly puke. It looks like he hasn't had a bath in about 6 months, and he has a thick beard that also stored an additional pint of vomit. So the cop is standing over us, Neil is doing a line, and I'm setting up the tube. I ask the cop if he can do CPR for us, while we set up. He looks me dead in the eye and says "no." "Excuse me," I asked. "No," he said again. Neil had to stop me from getting stupid with this cop. He told me not to bother, if they did CPR for us it was a courtesy and not a duty. At least we got to work this guy, even if he wasn't coming back. And to this day, I still think about what a piece of shit I thought that cop was.

So now we're parked by a church on One–Two–Seven and Lenox, as the job comes over. "18–Young…One–Four–Three and Riverside Drive, for the cardiac arrest." Neil tells me, "four arrests in a row is unusual, even for this unit," which has a rep for being one of the busiest in the city. He calls up the job on the KDT, as we travel to the sight. "This should be interesting," he says. The KDT states young male, cardiac arrest in the trunk of a car, PD requesting.

When we get there we see ESU has already popped the trunk. The smell is apparent from fifty feet away even in the open daytime air. It turns out this kid has been missing 3 weeks, and they just found his car four blocks away from his residence, illegally parked. The car had about thirty parking tickets on the windshield, and about 10 of those big yellow stickers that sanitation puts on the windows, stating "because you are illegally parked, this street could not be cleaned today." How's that for on the ball? Anyway, this kid had been cut up into 4 separate pieces, with a chainsaw or something, and was seal-a-mealed in Saran Wrap, then left in the trunk of his vehicle. Needless to say, this was a good crime scene. I couldn't understand, how nobody could smell the stench emanating from his vehicle, for the last three weeks—anyway, it was my first lesson in never fuck the Dominicans for drug money.

After that, we just did a couple of uneventful transports. And when I was travelling home, I was thinking, wow, every time I think my life sucks, I see something that that straightens my head right the fuck out.

The next time I worked with Neil was another very eventful tour. I particularly remember this day because I got my first pediatric save. It wasn't Neil's first, but he's already been a medic over nine years.

The morning started slow and we actually got to gas up he rig and get breakfast before we even got a job. Our first one hit about 8:15 in the morning. "18–Young…One–Two–Two and Douglas for the unconscious." Neil saw on the KDT that it stated four-year-old male, unconscious in the bathtub. Neil was driving, and I think he made that rig hit warp-6 in getting there.

We found a four-year-old kid supine, on the floor of the bathroom. His parents were both panic stricken. The kid was in respiratory arrest, and was cyanotic around his lips. He had been taking a shower with his dad. According to his hysterical mother, he slipped backwards in the tub, and slammed his head on the faucet. He also appeared to have aspirated some of the water. He had a weak brachial pulse, about 150, and absent breath sounds. I quickly measured him up for a tiny oral airway. I measured from his earlobe, to the outer edge of his lips. The kid accepted the airway, which I knew was a bad sign. I really hoped for an immediate gag reflex. Anyway, Neil was setting up a 4.5 ET tube, and I started to hyperventilate him. To my surprise, the kid started to gag on the airway. I removed it quickly and continued to bag him. We didn't even need to intubate him. We immobilized him inside a KED, and transported him to Harlem hospital, where he ended up fully recovering.

I loved this job, and I still tell my kids about it when they're about to get wild in the bathtub. Neil told me I did well, and it really meant a lot to me because I knew my evolution as a medic was coming along. The fact that I was able to stay calm and focused, while everything was turning to shit around us, was as important as the actual patient care itself.

So, it's a Monday morning, and between the job and the childcare, the bureaucracy and the mandates, I'm feeling like every minute of every day is Monday morning. I tell people, I think I'm functionally insane. I like working with Neil and Sarge, but the commuting on days is kicking my ass. November is here, the weather is starting to get colder, and that means flu season. An endless procession of bullshit taxi jobs that overwhelm our resources. Every asshole with a sniffle and congestion is a shortness of breath with chest pain according to our wonderful phone triage system. No one around here seems to have medical insurance, or a family doctor, but everyone has MediCard. We're used as a taxi service, and the ER is flooded with runny noses. I'm noticing that the nurses are as burnt as the EMT's and medics. And why not? I can't count how many real jobs I've missed because I've got to play nursemaid and mommy for Hector's fever. I think how many people's lives have been effected by waiting an extra 10 to 15 minutes during a real emergency, because all the units are tied up on the sniffles.

I still care about people. I want to do a good job, but I'm constantly tired now, and it's making me pretty snappy. So I'm working with Sarge. We get a typical bullshit job. Thirty-five-year-old female, difficulty breathing. We get into the elevator, which I now refer to as vertical urinals. There is so much piss in this elevator that it's bringing tears to my eyes, and my feet are sticking to the floor. I'm telling Sarge, "NY is a wonderful place. Where else can you smell the urine of 25 different nations, in one elevator?" Anyway, he's telling me "really how long will it be before a person is in an apartment, that they got to go in the corner of an elevator?" So we get out on our floor, and we're leaving wet footprints down the hall. We get to the door, and a woman lets us in. Sarge asks politely, "who's the patient?" The lady tells us she is, and she's been sick for three days, but she feels worse today. We ask her if she can go to her doctor, or the clinic, cause there's not much we or the ER will be able to do for her. She tells us she was at Columbia yesterday, and they just sent her home with some antibiotics, so she wants to go to St. Luke's instead.

We explained to her that the medicine is going to take a few days to work and she's not going to die. But we might have well been talking to the doorknob. She tells us that we have to take her where she wants to go, because her taxes pay our salaries. This would be true if she had a job in the past 15 years. So anyway, we take her over to St. Luke's which is packed, and go back into service for the next ungrateful, lifesucking, welfare vampire.

We get another job. "18–Young," the radio snarls…"One–Four–Eight and Bradhurst for the trauma." I'm thinking good, not another dif breather, maybe it will be a real job. Fat chance. We get to the scene, and it's a 25-year-old woman with a bloody nose. I mean, barely bleeding, maybe a few drops on a napkin. I ask her if she really wants to go to the hospital for this, and she does. She believes that by going to the hospital, it will give her a case to sue her boyfriend, who just smacked her. I said I would take her over to Harlem Hospital, but that she would sit a few hours for nothing. It didn't matter, she wanted the ride.

I said, "ma'am, I don't want to sound like I have an attitude or any-thing, but how would you feel if your mother, or someone you really loved was dying and we couldn't get to them because we're tied up with your bloody nose. She didn't miss a beat when she told us, "well I guess they'll just have to send another one." At this point I couldn't even begin to explain to her that there was no other one. We were the only unit in that area. So we just transported her, and I thought, well at least she walks.

So the next day I wake up at 5 am to begin my day. My kids are already awake and starting their day. I look out the window onto my street and I see it's fucking pouring out. I have a small river running down my driveway, and I'm thinking I'd like to go back to sleep—for about a hundred years. I walk into my bathroom to take a piss, but my daughter is already in there. She's toilet trained now, so of course she's standing over the toilet stirring up her lump of shit with the plunger like she's making soup.

I know this is why they have gun control in NY. If the cops hadn't taken all of my guns a couple of years ago, I probably would have put one in my head and been someone else's good job.

So, I do 2 miles an hour, all the way down the Staten Island Expressway, to cross the $7 bridge. I continue to crawl down the Brooklyn-Queens expressway, and cause I'm really late now, I pay another $3.50 shakedown, to go through the Brooklyn-Battery tunnel instead of the bridge into Manhattan, which is free, but its always a parking lot up there. I make decent time through the tunnel, but then on the FDR Drive, I'm stuck again. I really could have walked to work faster today.

As I finally get up to about 23rd Street on the drive, I see that 13 X-ray has started their day, with an upside down Impala that's taking out the left and center lanes of the northbound FDR. Well at least I got a good excuse I thought, when I get to work an hour and a half late. I'm still crawling up the drive, and at 96th Street there's another MVA. It looks like nothing more than allstateitis, but it's enough to set me back another half-hour.

So I get to work at almost 9:00. My lieutenant rips my asshole open a little wider. Jimmy, the lieutenant on the desk is really a good guy. He's very fair, but he's an absolute straight arrow, company man. No excuse in the world is good enough for not having the unit in service on time. He tells me if I need to watch the weather channel and wake up earlier, that's what I need to do. So Young is already in service without me. Instead, I'll work with Sophie on 19–Victor. Sophie is the hardest working woman I ever met in my life. She's a tough stocky German woman, who speaks with a thick Bavarian accent. She's over 50 and a grandmother, and I think half these motherfuckers we transport should be ashamed of themselves. I mean we have 30-year-old unemployed males telling her their sob stories, for the past fifteen years, expecting her to carry them down 3 flights of stairs, then wipe their asses for them, before we taxi them to the ER for bullshit.

Sophie knows what I've been going through. She's real nice to me, and knows how hard I'm trying to make everyone happy. She teaches me that most of the skells I work with are exactly that. Bullshitter's who talk better than they produce. She tells me, she'll work with me any day and that I just need to hang in there. Concentrate on all the good medics you work with and all the good things we're doing out here.

One thing is clear though. She's in charge, and I'll have to follow her lead. I really don't mind, cause she knows her shit upside down, and does the right thing even if it's inconvenient. I respect this very much, and I really have come to enjoy and look forward to working with her.

Our first job that morning is a little old lady about 75-years old. This patient is clearly stroked out. She's paralyzed on her right side. She can't talk to us, and she's incontinent of urine and fecal matter. She's drooling, and we can tell, she's been like this probably all night, until her family found her this morning. Anyway Sophie cancels our backup before they even get there. She tells Central we'll be on the scene, extended patient care for a while. I follow her lead and while assuring her family we're going to take care of her, we start to clean the patient up. I wiped the drool off her chin, and I hold her good hand for a little while. Sophie asks the family for a pot of warm water and a towel. She then proceeds to clean this woman up like she was her own mother, for the next ten minutes. She delicately wrapped her up in blankets, and wrapped a clean towel over her head like a kerchief. I thought Sophie made this patient look like Mother Theresa. We took her down to the rig, and she asked me if I would drive this job. I understood, and was more than happy to do this. On the way to CPMC, I was thinking this is super medic. No glory, no impossible tube, just do the right thing for everybody, unconditionally. Anyone who ever said anything about Sophie I knew was out with me.

So we leave CPMC, I'm thinking how one job can show a person's true characteristics. We're about to get coffee, when we hear a big one go over. Central sent a BLS unit over to One–Four–Three and Edgecombe, for a confirmed shot. It was Rona and Amber, two really good EMT's.

Sophie got on the air, and offered to back them up. We were put on the job, and arrived on the scene at the same time as 18–Bravo, the BLS unit. We got out of the rig, and it was raining so fucking hard now, that the drops were coming down sideways. We see in the concrete stairwell this 22-year-old male all contorted and laying face down on the stairs. He had been shot in the back of the head, and I was watching his blood spiral down the drain, as I selfishly thought, "they couldn't wait another 20 minutes for the rain to slow down before they did this." Anyway, me and the three females, got him in the scoop and on the rig, in about 90 seconds. We got to work all four of us cluttered in the back of the rig. Rona did CPR, while Sophie hit two 16-gauge IV's in this guy. Amber was suctioning him out for me, but the blood was coming out faster than we could get it. She continued to try to keep his throat clear for me as the blood bubbled out of his mouth. I set my tube, and went in with a Mac-4. I saw the esophagus, I wasn't able to see the trachea, but I knew where I didn't need to be. So I took the tube, and aimed high. This was my first blind tube. Sophie confirmed it was good and asked Rona to drive.

Rona asked dispatch to notify hospital 07 (Harlem), we were coming in with a shot, ALS on board. We worked real hard for this guy. Amber did CPR, Sophie put blood-pressure cuffs around the trauma bags, and got two liters of fluid in him real fast as she pumped them up. I continued to maintain the airway and hyperventilate, as Rona brought the rig up to sub-light speed. We got to Harlem hospital, and I was trying to work the tube and keep the Jell-O, which was the back of this kids head, together with a multi-trauma dressing, as Amber rode on the bar of the stretcher doing CPR. All of this was to no avail, which by now I had come to expect. The kid was pronounced dead shortly after our arrival. I thought in typical selfish terms, at least there was no family around that I had to talk to.

I figured something else would happen real soon, that would get my mind off the site of someone's blood running out of their head, and spiraling around the drain in a downpour. This was the kind of job that made you wish for the aggravation of some dope fiend on the 6th floor, or cleaning up your kids shit-soup at 5:15 am.

We were out of service for a while cause we had extensive BBP to do, and we still needed to restock. When I was mopping out the rig, Sophie came back with some fried rice and some sodas for us. She said lunch was on her, and she wouldn't take any money from me, even though I tried to stick a couple of dollars in her pocket. She told me if I didn't shut up and eat I would piss her off. So I thanked her for the food, and we went back in service.

I was talking to this guy Sy, who was the mayor of the station. He was out sick for an extended period of time, and hadn't been on a unit for a while. He lived right around the corner from the station, so he was there most of the time. He told me he was hearing good things about me, and after work if I wanted to come over to the loading dock, and drink with the boys, I was welcome to. I told him I would, and I was looking forward to it. Except that at 3:00 I got mandated for the evening tour, and had to work with Steve on 18–Young. So my initial hangout day got put on hold.

I knew Steve a little from passing, and having polite conversation. He was low-key and a genuinely nice person. I was tired and cranky, but I knew he would go out of his way to make it an easy afternoon for me, and I appreciated this. Besides, it had finally stopped raining and I thought the EMS god was through lifting his leg on me for today. Not quite. I was talking with Steve about the shooting earlier. He told me it was a shame the way people treated each other, and that most people were fortunate not to know what happens out here. So we're talking a little more when the radio tells us, "18–Young…you have an assignment, Henry Hudson Parkway, under the George Washington Bridge for the MVA." So we're extended from our area. It's only a little before dinnertime and traffic is still pretty heavy. We're having a hard time getting across the city, and we hear PD on the radio asking for a rush. When we get to the scene, there's an upside down car. The cop says, "the kid is still inside, and he looks bad." I crawl down on the cold wet pavement, and my heart falls into my stomach. It was a kid no older than 19, apparently he wasn't wearing a seatbelt, and when the vehicle flipped, the side of his head had been impaled on the rear-view mirror.

I probably would have been better off never seeing this job, cause almost every time I get in my car, I think about this kids brains on the interior roof of the vehicle. We got the kid extricated with ESU. He was clearly dead. The only way he was coming back was if Jesus Christ himself was coming down to work him. We transported him to CPMC, where he was pronounced. I was really fucked up now, and Steve knew it. I was almost crying when I told him, I just want to fuckin' go home already. So Steve asked for a patrol supervisor to meet us at the hospital, and our unit was put out of service. When I got to my car in the parking lot, I sat behind the wheel about 45 minutes with my key in the ignition, before I finally turned it on. I drove home, and when I got there I was real snappy. I promptly started a fight with my wife, and told her to "get the fuck away from me." She didn't deserve this, and couldn't begin to understand the kind of day I had. I was still so upset I locked myself in the bathroom, and was coughing until I vomited. I never came out that night, and I eventually fell asleep on the bathroom floor for a few hours. Guess what, I still had three more days to work, before my pass days would come.

I got back to work the next day, and immediately put in a hardship, to go back on overnights. My wife was getting fucked-up at her job, because we were both working days, and we didn't have anyone to watch our kids. I was told by the lieutenant that my request would be granted, but it would take a few days to get approved.

So I went into service with Sarge that day. He knew I was still fucked up from the day before, and he treated me to a coffee and a ham-and-egg sandwich, before we got a job. I didn't feel like working today, and it would have been all right with me if we just skelled-out the whole tour. This wasn't going to happen, though. 18–Young never sleeps, and although I begged the EMS god for an easy day, my prayers went unanswered.

My first job that day came over as an unconscious trauma in the street. The KDT told us unconscious female, on a hundred and forty-fourth and Hamilton Place. So we get on the scene, and there's this woman laying in the street, next to two parked cars. She's busted up pretty good, but she's not unconscious. I'm thinking her voice sounds really rough for a woman, but I still don't suspect anything, because she's pretty slinkily dressed, and I can clearly see that she's got fairly large breasts. So we put her on a board and in the bus. Sarge is talking to her, and she's telling us how this guy that picked her up, punched her in the face, and pushed her out of his jeep, while it was still moving. So I'm at the top and Sarge is at the bottom. I'm doing a blood pressure, and Sarge is cutting her dress off. All of the sudden I hear Sarge say in a real high voice, "Oh my God." Well it turns out she had this real skimpy little see-through underwear, which barely covered a penis about 10 inches long. Sarge was turning red, and I couldn't believe how faked out we were. Obviously, the guy who did this must have been faked out too. Anyway this person is looking at Sarge and asks him, "are you gay?" Well Sarge is a professional and although he's blushing he politely says, "well you know I try to stay happy at all times." So I can't contain myself. I'm laughing my ass off as he asks, "no, I mean are you homosexual?" Sarge looks back and says, "you know if you weren't my patient we would have to throw down now."

So needless to say, Sarge drove and I rode in the back. The whole day, I didn't let him live this down, and I was kidding him that I got the number for him, and put it on the ACR. So the day goes on, and I'm on an up in my manic-ness. I still laugh occasionally during the course of our tour, and Sarge knows why.

We get a street job, and it's a regular, this woman Cynthia, who every time she gets some money, she overdoses on heroin. Today she decided to OD in Taco Bell, on a Hundred and Thirty-third and Lenox. She's really out cold, as we get her on the rig. Sarge does the line, while I'm ventilating her. He blows the first shot, cause she's got like no veins left. So he gives her 2 mg of Narcan intramuscularly in the bicep. She's still out cold, and on the second attempt he hits a line in what we call the Junkie-vein. This is the vein on the underside of the forearm and it's always there because they can't see it, to shoot in. So he pushes dextrose, thiamin, and 2 more mg of Narcan through the IV. Now she wakes up, and she's pissed. I think we must have thrown her into instant withdrawal, because she's sitting up on the stretcher and calling me every four-letter word ever spoken. Suddenly, she pukes what looks like five pounds of bean burrito, all the fuck over me. I'm trying to clean myself, but this woman is going wild. I tell Sarge, just get her to the fucking ER, which is only three short blocks away. We get her out of the rig, and another unit that was there helped Sarge bring her in, while I was trying to get the puke out of my hair, and off of me. I went back to the station, and let me tell you, Sarge couldn't wait to get back to me. He starts belly laughing so fucking hard, I thought he was going to have a seizure. He says, "if I knew you were going to get a Harlem baptism, I would have invited a crowd," as he picks a kidney bean out of my eyebrow. Then he tells me, "you know Danny, I really feel for you, but you know how things are." I kiddingly told him to suck my dick, but that someone else might be jealous. Then we went out of service, extensive BBP. I was lucky I had a spare uniform in my locker, and after a quick shower and change, I came back to the unit. The rest of the day, everyone in the station made the sign of the cross, and laughed as they went by me.

CHAPTER 6

I'm still on days, but I was told by the captain that I'd go back on nights at the beginning of the month. This is great news cause I'm going to get to work with Jason regularly on 18–Young, midnight to 8 am. Our other partner will be Rod. He's the senior guy on the unit. He's one of the best medics at the station, and he's also a nurse. He's highly intelligent and very outspoken. So naturally, he's labeled a malcontent. Jason likes Rod a lot, and he lets me know that he thinks we're all going to get along fine, and he can't wait for me to get on the unit with them. They had been working with Robin, which I already know is torturous. She's been given a permanent vacation, and from what I'm told, she went to Barcelona, which as far as I'm concerned, still wasn't far enough away. I remember Rod describing working with her "is like your clothes are too tight, and bugs are crawling all over you, while the whole time, you have jock itch and a bad stomach virus." I told him, I'd rather be in that situation, than working with her. Anyway, the holiday season is coming, and I can't wait for the month to end. I'm working with Brendan on this day, cause Neil banged out. Brendan is real pissed because he got mandated, and he has to work with me. We still haven't ever worked together, and I'm determined to show him I'm a good guy and a good medic. So he tells me, he's working with me under protest, and I better not fuck with him today. I let him know that I really don't give a shit what he thinks and I'll prove him wrong for myself and not for him. So we're off to a good start aren't we, I thought, as we left the station to go save some lives and make a difference out here.

Our first job is One–Five–Three and Bradhurst for the stat epp. This is supposed to be a continuous seizure. We know that 99 out of a hundred times the job that comes over as a stat epp is nonsense, and probably never was even a seizure to begin with. It turns out these four guys about 40 or so, were drinking in the park all morning. So when one of them runs out of money, or becomes a pain in the ass, they just go over to a payphone, call 911, and tell the operator, someone had a seizure. So then EMS is sent, and there's one less set of lips around the bottle, as we scrape up the intox and take him to the hospital to get fed and take a nap. We'll probably pick this same guy up again tomorrow, which brings me into our next job that day—The legendary Levi, who also comes over the radio as an alleged seizure. We're sitting in the bay at Harlem hospital, we go available, and the radio chimes "8–Young…One–Four–O and Lenox for the stat epp." Brendan knows who we're going to get, before he even acknowledges that we're 63. He knows Levi's birthday, address, and even social security number by heart. Levi actually lives in the park, on a hundred and fortieth and Lenox. Any time it rains, gets cold, or he just wants to eat, he calls 911, and tells dispatch, he had a seizure. He then gets a $525 taxi ride to go four blocks, over to the hospital and crash out for a few hours. (Did you know an ambulance ride costs the taxpayers $525?) Anyway, Levi is transported, every day, no joke. Sometimes he's even transported 3 times a day. Everybody who has ever worked at Station 18, has transported Levi at least a half a dozen times.

He's actually a pretty funny and sociable guy, and I don't mind doing Levi at all, cause he always walks to the rig for me. He always greets me the same way. "Hey man, what's happening?" I don't even get a chance to answer him before he continues, "gimmee a cigarette man, you got a quarter for me?" I tell Levi I'll give him a cigarette at the ER, because I know he'll try to light it on the rig. And if I give him one before he gets on, he'll smoke it before he moves for us. On this particular day, Levi summoned the unit, because he had gotten a bill from EMS for

$207,000. I'm not kidding—$207,000! Anyway, he's vintage, drunk off his ass. He's showing me and Brendan this bill, and he's telling us, "I ain't gots no two thousand seven dollars, for no fucking EMS." Brendan lights his cigar stub, as he stares in the bill in disbelief. He's laughing now, and he's telling Levi the bill is for two hundred and seven thousand dollars, and maybe he should stop calling EMS. Levi is laughing, and he tells Brendan, "say what, give me a quarter, B." He then continues, "you're the motherfucker who brought me down to St. Vincent's last night." "I had to walk all the way back." "I hads no money, and passed 9 liquor stores on the way up." Brendan says to him, "Well I see you got back safely, and you must have found some money, when you got to the tenth one." So Levi steps onto the rig for us, and when we got to the emergency room, I gave him 2 cigarettes and a dollar. And inside myself, I was actually grateful for Levi today, because it actually broke the ice between Brendan and I.

So after we do Levi, Brendan is standing by the rig. He lights his cigar stub, and I'm thinking, "man, he sure gets his money's worth out of those things." "He's probably had that one since 3 am." So we get a job all the way up in Washington Heights. It states "unknown condition." It turns out this guy Miguel that works with us as an EMT, is smelling something really foul, coming from an apartment in his building. Well Miguel is a veteran, and the smell of death is familiar to him. When we get to the scene, the cops are already there. Miguel tells Brendan, "this guy is crazy, and no one's seen him in about two weeks." Brendan knows something's up inside this apartment, and when no one answers the door, he calls ESU over the radio, so the door can be taken. Anyway, when ESU gets there, Brendan knows its show time. He goes into this pouch on his belt, and pulls out a small jar of Vicks Vapor Rub. I don't know what he's going to do with this, but I soon find out. He takes out a big gob of goo, and starts smearing it in his moustache. He lights his cigar stub, and steps back, as ESU takes the door. The door pops open, and an overwhelming stench of death bombards the hallway. Cops start coughing. I'm about to puke, and Brendan walks right into the apartment and says "Lucy, I'm home," in his best Cuban accent. I come in behind him, and we see a guy, who hung himself in a doorway, with a long orange extension cord. He's been there enough time, that his head is ready to pop off. So I ask Brendan if I can borrow some of his Vicks. He saw I was as green as our corpse, and he let me use it. It still didn't matter. Even the menthol smell wasn't enough, and I went into the bathroom and vomited. After that, I always carried Vicks and a big smelly cigar, and I vowed I would never go near another DOA without my vital equipment.

When we got down to the rig, Brendan gave me a couple of 4x4 bandages, to get the Vicks out of my mustache. And he told me, "I guess there was something I could teach you after all." I knew I would like Brendan, but I couldn't let onto this yet. It was going to be a long hard road to earn his respect, and being a puking madman, I hadn't helped my cause. We let Central know that we had an eighty-three, left with PD. It was almost noon, and we would probably only do one more job before Brendan took the rig back and went out of service, overtime personnel.

We're up on One–Five–Eight and B'way, and we're eating some fried chicken wings. Brendan starts dipping these wings in some death sauce, that I knew was going to burn him a new asshole. I took my wings, and I said maybe I shouldn't eat, cause I know that we're going to get a job as soon as I take a bite. Well, sure as shit, we get one. Central asks our location, then sends us to Post and Dykeman for a dif breather. We get to the scene and we walk up four flights of stairs to the apartment. I ask B, "doesn't anyone get sick on the first floor around here?" I knew he was tired and this job had bullshit written all over it. When we get in there's like 20 people in this hermetically sealed apartment. It was about 35 degrees outside, but it was about 95 in this place. We were in about 10 seconds, and were led into the living room, where this 300-pound woman was lying on the couch with a cold rag on her head going "I…Yi…Yi, I…Yi…Yi, I…Yi…Yi," holding her chest, and sounding like a broken record on 78. We try to get her to talk to us, but all she would say is, "I…Yi…Yi." Brendan looked over to me and said, "status hispanicus." He had seen this type of job a hundred times. We talked to one of her sons, and he told us his mother didn't like her daughter's new boyfriend. So now we know she's trying to make her feel guilty by calling the whole damn family there, and acting like she's having a heart attack.

We assessed her needlessly, and found her to be warm, BP of 130/76 and a rate of 76. I told Brendan I'd seen better performances out of Fred Sanford, as he asked the woman to come with us. He told her sons we were going to take her over to CPMC. Well the sons are telling us, she's sick, she can't walk, you gotta carry her. Well I'm thinking, yeah, I'll carry her fat ass down four flights of stairs, for this bullshit, when pigs fly. Brendan is not giving an inch, as he tells them, "sir, it's my job to know when someone needs to be carried." "We think your mother is going to be fine." "We only want her to go to the hospital to get checked out and make sure." I thought this was real diplomatic, as she got off the couch and walked down to the rig for us.

When we got to the hospital, the triage nurse summed this up as usual nonsense, and sent her to the waiting area, where she promptly walked out of the hospital. We went out of service and back to the station. I told Brendan before we left, that I was glad I worked with him, and that I hope I didn't make him too miserable. He said I wasn't as bad as he had heard, and he farted as he left the station. I was real glad we were done before those chicken wings started kicking in. I still had two hours left in my tour, but there was no one there to work with me. Jimmy was the lieutenant on the desk that day, and we bullshitted, and I did some paperwork for him. It only took about 15 minutes, and when I was done, Jimmy told me I could fill out a request for leave sheet and go home. He told me when I got home safe, to call the station and let him know. Then he would tear up the sheet, so I wouldn't be charged for the time. I thought this was really cool, especially because he didn't have to do this for me. I beat the traffic home, and thanked the EMS god for an easy day as I called the station.

CHAPTER 7

So Neil is in today. As much as I like him and Sarge, I'm thankful I've only got a couple of days left before I go back on nights. Our day starts out like any other. A bullshit job before we even get the rig checked out, let alone a cup of coffee. By now I've learned, if I want coffee, I have to pick it up before I get to the station.

The voice of doom calls out, "8–Young…One–Two–Six and Douglas for the inbleed." Real inbleeds are rare, and usually very disgusting and messy. So I'm glad it's probably bullshit. Neil tells Central, "10–4, mark me 63, unchecked vehicle." We called the job up on the KDT, and it states, 26-year-old female, bleeding from rectum. So I'm thinking, yeah, my ass hurts too, but I ain't calling no fucking ambulance for it. Since an inbleed is a dual response, we got a BLS backup. After we enter the building, we get into this piss-stenched elevator, all of us together. Me, Neil, Alex and Joey (our backup), two cops, and a couple of firemen. When we assess the patient, we find out she's got hemorrhoids, I tell Neil, "this is great." "Two EMS units, a PD patrol vehicle, and a fire company for fucking hemorrhoids." "No wonder this fucking city is broke." Anyway, Alex can see I'm pissed and he pulls me on the side, and tells me that they'll take this job for us. I thanked him, and said I didn't have a protocol for the `roids, anyway. The firemen left shaking their heads, as if they weren't used to this either, by now. We let Central know we 84'd the patient to BLS, and went back in service. It didn't take long for another to hit. "8 Young," the overseer summoned. "One–Two–Two and Amsterdam for the cardiac arrest." Neil got pissed, this was 6 Willie's job. They had been out of service restocking for about 45 minutes. "I'm shocked," I told Neil, "6 Willie holding a signal—that's unheard of," I said sarcastically. We get to the building, and once again, we hike up the stairs to the apartment. This hysterical woman answers the door, yelling come in, come in, hurry. The problem was there was this tremendous sentinel of a German shepherd that wasn't going to let us enter unless we paid the toll with our flesh. So Neil is standing there telling her, "Ma'am, please come put the dog away. Please get the dog, so we can enter." The lady comes and grabs the dog by his neck, and pulls him into the kitchen. In the bathroom we find this middle-aged man in arrest. The toilet bowl is filled with bloody diarrhea, and it reeks. So as we drag him into the hall, so we can work, I flush the bowl. We get the monitor on and I'm setting up the tube, as it shows V-fib. So we got to shock him. We still have LifePak-5's, so we've got to use the paddles. Anyway, like a crazed hellhound, this animal comes tearing out of the kitchen, and is standing over the body snarling, and growling at Neil and me. I'll still never figure out how Neil stayed calm. He's calling out in a slow, low-key tone, "Ma'am, come get the dog." The woman is still in the kitchen, blind with fright. I'm on the other side of the body, and I'm whispering, "shock the dog. Shock the fucking dog!" Neil just says a little louder, "Ma'am, please come get the dog." Well the woman never heard him, but she did look back to see what we were doing. I heard her scream, "oh my God," as she ran in and grabbed the animal. We shocked this guy three times—200–300–360. On the third shock, he converted to sinus. Neil started a line, and we hit him with lidocane, then set up a drip. The sinus didn't last long, and he went flat-line on us. So now he's intubated, he's getting epi's and atropines, as we run fluid into him.

We get down to the rig, and he goes V-fib again. We shocked him three more times, back into flat-line. CPR'd him back to V-fib, and shocked him back to asystole. This pretty much continued all the way to St. Luke's. This patient didn't make it, and I was real upset that he didn't. We really left it all on the street for this guy. It was the first time I ever saw Neil sweat. But by now I was fully convinced, he was the best medic I had worked with up to that point. In the ER, I was covered in sweat, even though it was like 20 degrees out.

We're back at the station, and not in service yet. I'm still doing restock, and Neil is talking with Matt about the arrest we just did. I know Matt pretty well, and if you saw him you would think he was a pushover. He's real skinny, and never speaks, unless he has something important to say. Because Matt is so quiet and focused, people think he is weird. But I know he's just an elitist. He's deceivingly strong, and extremely smart. I remember Rod once telling me, Matt was voted most likely to go up in the bell tower with a rifle. Anyway, I really liked Matt, and I had worked well with him, but that's another story.

We hear 19–Xray get a job for a shooting on One Hundred and Thirty-fifth and Powell. They're a distance away, and let Central know this. Well like I said, we're still not done restocking, and our bags are still undone in the back of the rig. Neil gets on the air, and calls out, "Young—I'm right around the corner from that job. Put me on it." He tells me to jump in the front, but I'm already there, ready to rock again. Matt tells us to hurry up and go, and he'll talk to us later, as we're already rolling. It takes us literally less than thirty seconds to get to the scene. In the hall of the building, we see a sixteen-year-old kid shot once in the chest. There's a lot of blood on his shirt, but to my amazement, he's very alert, and talking to the cops. He's telling them he doesn't know the guy who did this, but everyone knows he's lying. Neil grabs the board, and I grab the trauma bag. We quickly get between the cops and the patient, and lay him on the board. I cut his shirt off, and I see a small hole, about the size of a dime, in the center of his chest, and no exit wound. Neil bangs a line in him before I even got a blood pressure. The kid is tearing the non-rebreather off his face telling me, "I don't need this shit, just take me to the fucking hospital." So we get him in the bus, and I'm thinking this kid is really tough, he's not even scared. I'm trying to get him to tell me who did this to him, but he just says "don't sweat me, man, I'm going to deal with it." We get him into the emergency room. The whole job happened so fast that they weren't even notified yet that we were coming. I'm telling Neil afterwards that I thought the kid would be OK, and he was really lucky, all things considered. Neil told me, "don't be so sure," and pointed out to me the fact that there was no exit wound was really bad.

Anyway, we finished up our tour a couple of hours later, and before I left I went over to the emergency room to check on the kid. I expected that they would tell me he was going to be OK. I was genuinely shocked, when the nurse told me sadly and quietly that he had died in the OR. Man, I was fucking pissed. The whole ride home, I was blasting my Metallica tape, Seek and Destroy, For Whom the Bell Tolls, and then Fade to Black. I smoked a big fucking joint going over the Verrazano Bridge, and thought, fuck this shit, I'm banging out tomorrow. I didn't though. I went back to start the whole fucking endless process again.

CHAPTER 8

So it's my last day, before I go back on nights. I'm looking forward to this, and I got three days off after today. I had worked on Thanksgiving, and it's the forth year in a row I had to do this. The way the schedule was working, I would also have to work Christmas, New Years and my birthday. I still haven't had a Christmas off since my kids were born, and this goes all the way back to the privates. Anyway, I'm working with Matt today, and it's fucking freezing out. There's some snow on the ground, and everything is really icy and slippery. I'm bitching to Matt about the schedule, but inside I know he doesn't want to hear it. I think he was grateful that we got a job, cause it would mean I would have to shut up for a while.

We get sent to a Hundred and Twenty-fifth and St. Nick, for the unconscious in the subway. We got backup on this job, and it's 18–Henry, a good EMT unit that's got a rep for really working hard. They're on the scene first, and they ask us for an ETA. We let them know we're right by the Apollo Theater, and we'll be there quick. So I hear Alex, over the air, tell us to keep it coming, cause this guy needs ALS. He also tells us to bring a board and a collar down. When we get to the scene, we find a middle-aged man, whom witnesses stated had slipped down the icy, concrete subway stairs. The three of us, me, Matt and Alex log rolled this guy onto the board, and Joey told me the guy had a hole in the back of his head that you could fit a teaspoon in. So Matt tells me, you got to work this guy on the fly, and I definitely agreed. We climbed out of the stairwell. Joey drove, and Alex was in the back with us. We started towards St. Luke's as Matt set up the lines. I set the tube, and Alex bagged him for us. We hit the lines and the tube, and the patient started to have a seizure, as we pulled up to the emergency room. The hospital was just getting the notification as we were coming in. They gave this guy Valium, and it broke his seizure. I still don't know if this patient lived, but I felt we were quick and efficient, and that we did a good job. This was just another way to start, I thought, as I changed the bloody sheet on my stretcher.

I knew Matt thought I was a wacko, so I figured I would play it up with him. I brought two coffees back to the rig, and I was singing in a slow methodical tone, "start your day with a DOA, do-dah, do-dah." Well Matt wasn't too amused. As usual he didn't say a word. He just gave me one of those crooked, are you out of your fucking mind, death stares. We got through the rest of the morning without anything eventful happening. I talked, and Matt tolerated me.

We got a job in the barrio, in the early afternoon, and it turned out to be another memorable one. "8–Young," the radio called. "One–Two–Two and Two, for the OB comp." These are usually nonsense taxi jobs, but not this time. We get to the scene, and it's one of those white hi-rise buildings over there. We have to walk all through the maze to get in. We get into the elevator. Just as the door closes, someone sticks his hand in and makes the door open. We're going up to the twenty-something floor, and this inconsiderate bastard, steps in and pushes the button for twelve. I'm thinking, you stupid scumbag, how would you feel if I was going to get your mother, and someone did that. Anyway, we get to the apartment, and this young Spanish woman is in labor, and her contractions are 10 seconds apart, or something stupid like that. I can't figure why she waited so long to call a bus, or just go to the hospital. In between screams, she tells us she's got to go to the bathroom. We know we can't let her go take a shit. I'm asking her if she can hold it, but she's already crowning. Matt doesn't think we can get her down to the elevator, let alone to North General or Met, and I agree. She's going to deliver, so

I'm saying to myself get your catcher's mitt ready, and Matt sets up the OB kit. All of a sudden with one big push, I get hit with this blast of exploding diarrhea, and the baby popped out. Matt clamped and cut the cord, while I suctioned the baby's mouth and nose, with the bulb syringe. We quickly cleaned and wrapped a beautiful healthy baby boy, and as the placenta delivered, our BLS backup finally arrived.

So we're down on the rig. Mommy is really happy, and I'm smiling my ass off. I looked over at her and I asked, "so what's his name?" She looked back at me and paused, and then said, "what's your name?" Well I'm feeling real full of myself now, and I proudly say, "my name is Danny." She pauses again, and then asks, "do you have any brothers?" I went from feeling like Tarzan, to Rodney Dangerfield, in half a second.

When we got back to the station, I told Matt I was going back on nights to work with Jason and Rod. I said I'll see you around, and he responded, "yeah, sooner than you think, cause I'm going on nights too." And he told me he was going on X-ray with Rich and Tom. I thought this was great, and he was happy, cause he liked both of them.

CHAPTER 9

Being back on nights is good for me. I'm working with people who I like, and who like me. I'm gaining a lot of credibility, and for the time being, I'm happy. Working with Jason is the best thing to happen for me. We're having a lot of laughs, and we're working like animals. We take pride in being the busiest unit in the city. Tom and Rich have given us permission to pick up all of their trauma and arrest jobs, and any other jobs that we want to pick up. We're working a Friday night on Young. The full December moon is large, and I'm superstitious. So I tell Jason, we're in for a hell of a night.

We get out of the box at midnight, and one of my buddies on BLS has been in service since 10. We hear over the air that they're going to One–Two–Two and Manhattan Avenue for a stabbing.

We knew the tour 3 guys weren't skells, so when they told us the bus was in good shape, we knew we could go immediately into service without a problem. I got on the air, and asked Central to put us on the back of 16–Charlie. We got to the scene of a chaotic street job. This kid about 17 was slashed across his cheek with a box-cutter. The initiation into a local gang was, you had to slash someone, we were told. This kid had a real clean, painless cut, but it bled like a son-of-a-bitch. He told us about 10 guys had run up to him, someone slashed his cheek, and they just kept running. He was real upset, because he was concerned he was going to have a nasty scar. There wasn't much we could do except bleeding control. We took him over to St. Luke's, and before we were ready to get back in service, we picked up a job on One–Four–O and St. Nicholas.

We heard X-ray get assigned a job for a jumper down at that location. We were coming out of the ER, when it came over the air. Tom told Central that he would be extended from his area. I knew he would be just a slight bit perturbed, at having to do this job in our area. So I got on the air, and told Central that we were 98 out of Luke's and we were closer. Tom was 87'd and he thanked me over the air. I knew we had stayed on his good side tonight, and Jason saw I was happy about this.

So there's a couple of good things about working the upper West Side. One of which is that our FM radio picks up 89.5 Seton Hall Pirate Radio just fine. We're zipping up St. Nick, and we're blasting Guns-n-Roses Welcome to the Jungle, as we arrive on the scene. We find a really decrepit looking, withdrawn, 75 pound female, sprawled and mangled on the sidewalk. She's screaming in pain at the top of her lungs, and you can't even touch her without getting your eardrums punctured.

So as the story goes, this guy came home and saw that all his money was gone. He later found his wife, or whoever she was, out on the fire escape smoking crack (mind you it's like 15 degrees out). So he did what any self-respecting man would do—he tossed her off the third floor fire escape. Well he was going to do time for this, and I thought this place is fucking insanity. We tried our best to immobilize her. She had bilateral femur fractures and was busted up real good. It turns out she was also three months pregnant.

We took her to Harlem Hospital, and although I was just about deaf from her screams of agony, I was able to bang a line in her. I knew the aggravation of this job was nothing compared to what would have happened if Tom and Rich had been forced to pick it up.

We take about 10 minutes in the emergency room to get our brain cells back, and go into service again. We've only been working about an hour and a half, but we had already banged out two good jobs. I walked across the street to the station, where I talked to Brendan for about two minutes. He was coming into service on a 1 am unit, and he still hadn't finished checking his rig, but Central was trying to give him a job in the

Polo grounds, for an unconscious. Jason saw us talking, and came over and asked if I wanted to do the job. I said I would. I called Central over the air, "8–Young." Central answered, "Young…go." I told them, "put us on Victor's job, we'll take it." We go 63, and see on the KDT, unconscious male, in the hallway, up on the 24th floor.

Well it turns out only one of the three elevators in the building is working. There's about 15 people in the lobby and the smell of drugs is so strong, I'm thinking if I got piss tested now, I would probably be positive for crack. So the vertical urinal finally gets down, and every other person is asking us where we're going. They almost always catch an attitude with you when you let them know you're not allowed to tell. Anyway, we get in the elevator with all our equipment. I can't put it down, because of the piss puddle on the floor. Anyway, everyone else piles into the elevator with us. No one thinks twice about hitting all their buttons. We hit 24, but other people hit 6,10,14,19, etc. It takes about 10 minutes to get up to our floor, where we find an intoxicated, unconscious man, in a thick yellow puddle of vomit, with a half eaten chicken wing in the center of it. So we push the button for the elevator, to come back. In the time it takes to get to us, we hit a line, gave him dextrose, narcan and thiamin, got him packaged for transport, and were still waiting for the fucking elevator. As it turns out, someone near the top hit all the buttons, and this fucking thing stopped on every floor on the way down. We put him in the rig, and Jason stayed in the back, while I headed us over toward Columbia.

When we went in service again, we headed over to One–Seven–Eight and B'way, to eat at a 24-hour Spanish restaurant over there. We were eating our cubanos, which I believed tasted even better at 2 in the morning. We hear a job for an MVA on the George Washington Bridge. The radio calls, "19–Victor…west bound upper level, for the overturned vehicle." We don't even tell Central we're going. We're right under the bridge as it is. So in forty-five seconds, I get on the air, and I say, "8–Young…show me on the scene of Victor's job." Sure enough, the car is upside down in the center lane. The guy had already crawled out, and he was the only person in the car. Amazing as it sounds, he was fine. He had been wearing a seatbelt, and I guess that's the reason he didn't even have a scratch on him. He tells us he doesn't need to go to the hospital. I said, "I would tell you God bless you, but I think he just did."

By now, Brendan's unit shows up and he's acting pissed cause I buffed his job. Anyway, this guy was going kind of fast, in the left lane. The wind was blowing so hard, my nuts had crawled up into my pelvic cavity as the gales tore my sac off. He said he lost concentration for just a second, because a gust of wind had caused him to sideswipe the guardrail. He panicked and cut the wheel back too fast, rolled his vehicle, then skidded on the roof about 500 feet. The car was really fucked up, and this guy was not physically hurt at all. As a matter of fact, he wanted to RMA. I advised against it, and so did Jason, but he insisted he didn't want to spend all night in a hospital. We called for a patrol supervisor, who witnessed our refusal of aid. We then went over to the Jersey side, made our turn, and proceeded to cross our gateway of misery, back into paradise.

We're back in service about an hour, before we get another assignment. It's back down on a hundred and twenty-third street, on the West Side. It's another of our regulars, Otis. He's really nasty, and he's had a heart attack every night now for the past 7 or 8 years. Otis is as frequent a flyer as Levi. I asked in my most polite voice, because I didn't want to set him off, "how are you feeling tonight, sir, are you alright?" He snapped at me, "you all know how I am motherfucker, I'm ill." "Now take me over to the hospital, and don't ask me no questions, and don't be touching me either." So I did the only smart thing I could, I dumped him on my good buddy, and best partner, and I drove. Jason climbed out of the rig at St. Luke's, while I walked away to get a wheelchair. When I got back, he gave me a hard slap on the back, and said in a loud slow way, "buddy, tomorrow YOU'RE in the back with him."

We continue to be car service for the next few hours, and in the morning I was pretty ripe. I thought I was going to sleep with one eye today, and watch some college football with the other. But as it turns out, my daughter has other plans. I promised her we would do the Christmas tree.

So, when I went back to work that night, I was wiped out before I even got out of the parking lot. We were signing out our narcs, and Lieutenant Lardass told us we were getting a student. He was a Navy Seal doing his clinical rotations in Harlem, as part of a Special Forces medic program out of San Antonio. His name was Kenny, and he was a big likeable guy from West Virginia. He spoke with a slow drawl and we liked his accent as much as he liked ours. I like having students, and I was really glad to have someone to help with the carry-downs.

I'm determined to stay busy tonight, even though I'm really tired. We get a job fast. "One–Two–Eight and Morningside, for the unconscious." The KDT tells us, 68-year-old male, unresponsive, in bed. It also tells us cardiac, diabetic, and seizure history, as per female caller. I tell Ken, this sounds like a good job for you. It might even be an arrest. When we get up to the apartment, we're led into the bedroom, and this guy is laying in bed, wet, cold, gurgling respirations, and unconscious. Kenny does a blood pressure, and I start to bag him. Jason puts the monitor on, and he's in A-fib at 96 to 120. Ken tells us the BP is 200/100, and I point out the very swollen ankles as just another indicator. The lady gives us a baggie of drugs that contains digoxin, lasix, K-dur, tegretol, and aspirins, and she says his insulin is in the refrigerator. So Jason tells Kenny, "he's in pulmonary edema, and has probably burned up all his sugar." We let Ken do a line, an 18-gauge in the right antecubital, a good hit. We drew bloods for him, and then we let him push dextrose. Our patient starts to wake up a little, and the cookbook recipe continued. We pushed 80 mg of lasix, and then a hundred mg of thiamin. We explained why it wasn't necessary to give narcan, but Kenny already knew this. Besides, our patient was awake now. We gave him a nitro, and his breathing was still labored, and his pressure was over 190. We gave him another nitro, he was still having a lot of chest pain, so Jason gave him a third, as I got on the phone with medical control. After explaining the situation, I got an order for morphine, a baby aspirin, and repeats of nitro, every five minutes as needed, as long as blood pressure remained stable.

So we gave our patient 5 mg of morphine, and made him comfortable. His blood pressure was still over 160, and the monitor was still A-fib. We gave some more morphine, and down in the rig, gave a fourth nitro, and a last 5 mg of morphine. The patient said he felt fine at this time, as he chewed up the baby aspirin. Kenny thought we were great, and he couldn't believe this guy was in a coma, just 15 minutes ago. We took the patient to St. Luke's, where he thanked us and told the nurse we had taken good care of him. When we went back in service, I got a bagel and coffee over on One–Ten and B'way.

After restocking our narcotics, Ken was itching for another job, and Central didn't disappoint us. We didn't even finish our snack when we got sent to 3333 Broadway, for the altered mental status. So Ken's in the back of the rig looking forward through the square dividing hole, and asks what we've got. I told him, "it looked like no big deal, probably an intox on the street." We sped up Broadway; it was quick, straight two-minute run. Sure enough, we find a guy about 35, standing on the corner of a hundred and Thirty-fifth Street, disoriented and intoxed, spewing Spanish pro-fanities. He had been slashed up with a box-cutter pretty good, about four times along his neck and face, on both sides. There's a lot of blood all over this guy, and on the ground. Jason says, "our boys from the other night are hard at work again." And I explained to Ken about the slashing initiation.

We cleaned up our patient. We let Kenny drop an 18 in him, and push the coma cocktail of dextrose, narcan, and thiamin. It didn't do anything for our guy, but then we don't have an antidote for tequila in that mix. So we transported back down to Luke's.

We were back in service, and played car service for a couple of hours. One of these jobs was extremely annoying. We got a job for an asthma on One–Two–Eight and Lenox on the street. It turns out this fifteen-year-old girl, is on the corner with her boyfriend. She tells us its asthma, but it's not. She's got a fever and a cough with congestion, no wheezing, and she tells us it's cold, and she knew we would come faster, if she told the operator on the phone that she was having an asthma attack. So she's telling Jason, she's got to go to St. Luke's, because she lives over in that area. Well Jason is pissed, and I'm feeling that these are the jobs that really wear you down. He says to her, "you called 911 for an emergency, you need to go to the nearest hospital, which is Harlem." She tells him "no," and he responded that if she wanted to go to St. Luke's she should call Malcolm (the neighborhood car service). So she's getting uptight, and her boyfriend tells us he knows the law, and we've got to bring her where she wants to go. The sad thing is he's right, and I'm telling myself, damn, these kids already know how to play the system. So I say to Ken, "at least we're not carrying her." We drove to St. Luke's, and amazingly, she felt well enough not to even go into the emergency room, as she decided to walk up the remaining block to the building where she lived. I went into the ER to use the bathroom and wash up. While I was in there, I saw our diabetic, pulmonary edema patient, who we had brought in earlier. He was sitting upright and awake, speaking to his son, who had probably not gotten there too long ago.

As I moved on, I looked in on our slashing patient, and he was sleeping. His wounds turned out to be superficial enough, that no stitches were needed. They were bandaged over antibiotic ointment. I went out and told Jason, our patients were doing better, and we went back in service.

We drove up to our area, on the triangle where a Hundred and Thirty-sixth Street meets St. Nicholas Avenue and Edgecombe Avenue. We didn't get another job until after sunrise, and I had actually fallen out for a few minutes. Jason elbowed me awake, and informed me, we were going to be 63 to a seizure job, in the projects on One–Two–Six and Douglas. I noticed we would be going in for the change in about an hour, and I wasn't getting mandated today. I thought this looked like a good bullshit job, that we could bang out easy.

So we get to the building, and we're locked out. We can't even get in the hall to ring the bell. It's really cold, and this is very frustrating. I come up on the air, and I ask Central to please call back for entry. In about two minutes, our dispatcher informs us, that a lady will come down to let us in, and the patient was still having a seizure. So I'm getting real antsy. By now our backup and PD are all out here freezing. It took over five minutes for this elderly lady to get down to the lobby, and open the door for us.

We step into a small, used, vertical urinal and there's nowhere in the elevator you can step without getting urine on your shoes. We come to a tenth floor apartment, and find an elderly man, in just his pajama bottoms, sitting up against an uncovered radiator. He's seizing and unresponsive. There's a spilled bottle of dilantin next to him, and about forty pills are scattered on the black-and-white tiled floor. We move him off the radiator, and his neck and back are covered with second-degree burns, with huge blisters.

Alex prepared a sterile burn sheet with sterile water, and wrapped him up in it. We estimated he had been there at least thirty minutes, until his wife came out of the bedroom and found him. I inserted an oral airway, that was accepted, and bagged him, while Jason set up the tube and a line. I let Ken do the line, and I did the tube, while Jason got on the phone for a Valium order. When he got off the phone, the patient was wrapped and on a scoop stretcher, the line was secured, and Ken had already pushed the coma cocktail without any positive change. The patient was very hot, and still seizing after I had landed an 8.0 tube in him. I let Alex ventilate it, while confirming it clear bilaterally. Jason told me we had the Valium order, in increments of 5 mg, IV push, until the seizures subsided. We gave 5 mg, without a change, then let the student push the second 5 mg after he had observed the administration of the first dose. There was still no change, and we continued to breathe for our patient, as Jason and Kenny passed another 5 mg through the IV tubing and let it flush through. Our patient stopped seizing, and we brought him out to the hall, and waited for the elevator to come back.

The elevator was too small to put a stretcher in supine, so being that his blood pressure was 90/60, we decided that it would be better to put him in the elevator head-down, instead of head-up. This way, his heart and brain would be better perfused, as we continued to run fluid into him, and breathe for him. I was down on my knees in the elevator. My pants were wet, and I knew it hadn't been raining in here. The smell of urine was strong enough to floor me, and I thought it sucked that the guy's head had to be so close to this. The good thing was, if he lived he wouldn't remember it.

When we got down to the rig, we asked dispatch to notify hospital 07, that we would be there in 3 to 4 minutes. I let Kenny drop another line in him, on the bus, and I was happy he hit a 16. We went en route to Harlem hospital, and when we were done with our paperwork, Kenny was telling us that he thought we were amazing, and kicked ass tonight. I was physically exhausted, and wanted to get to the parking lot as soon as I could.

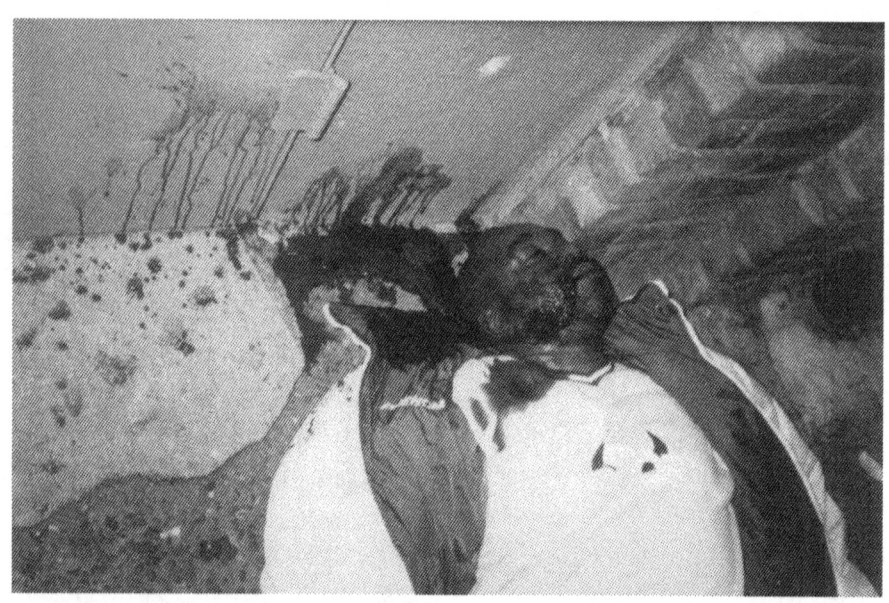

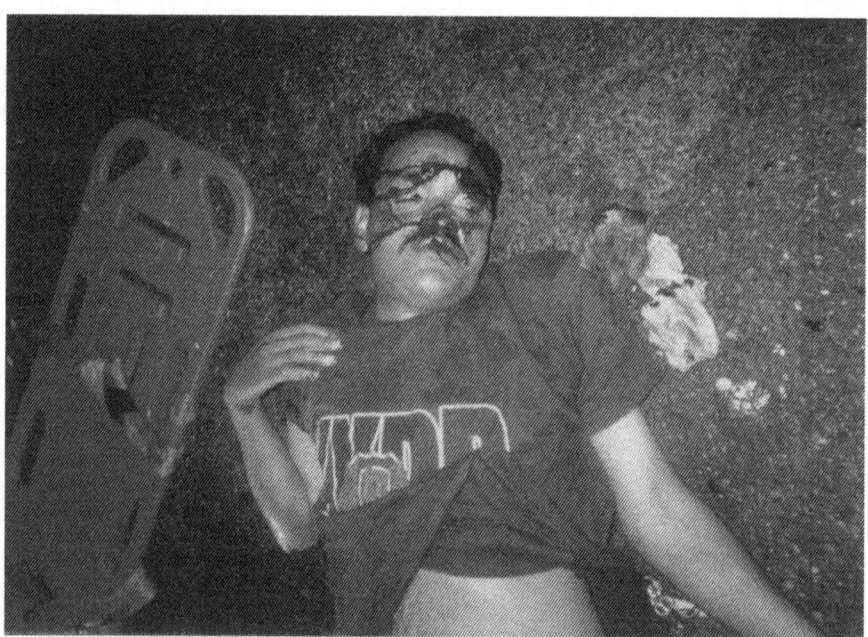

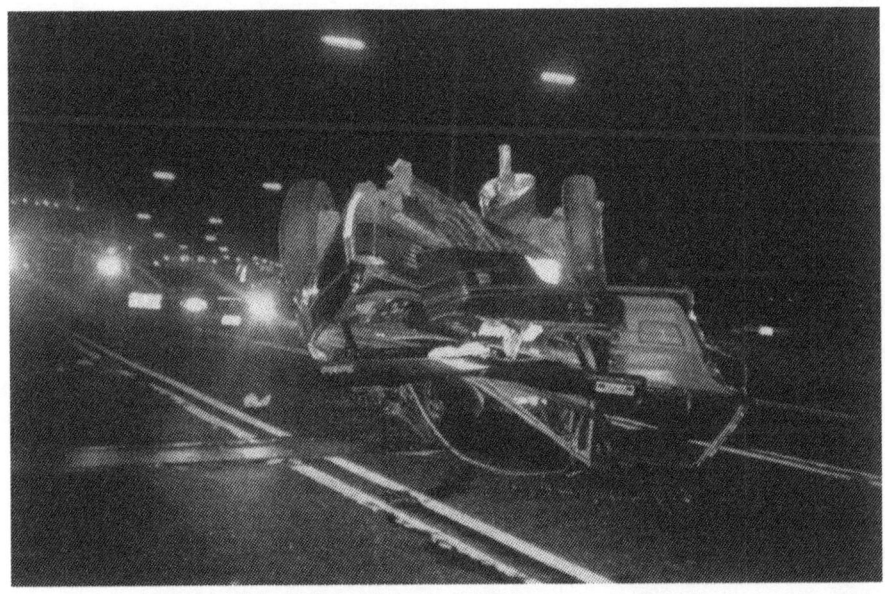

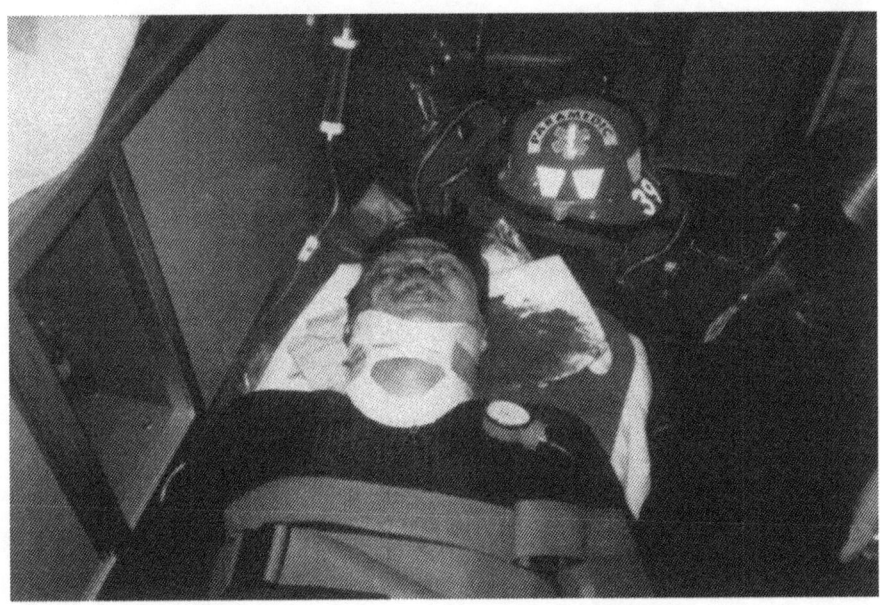

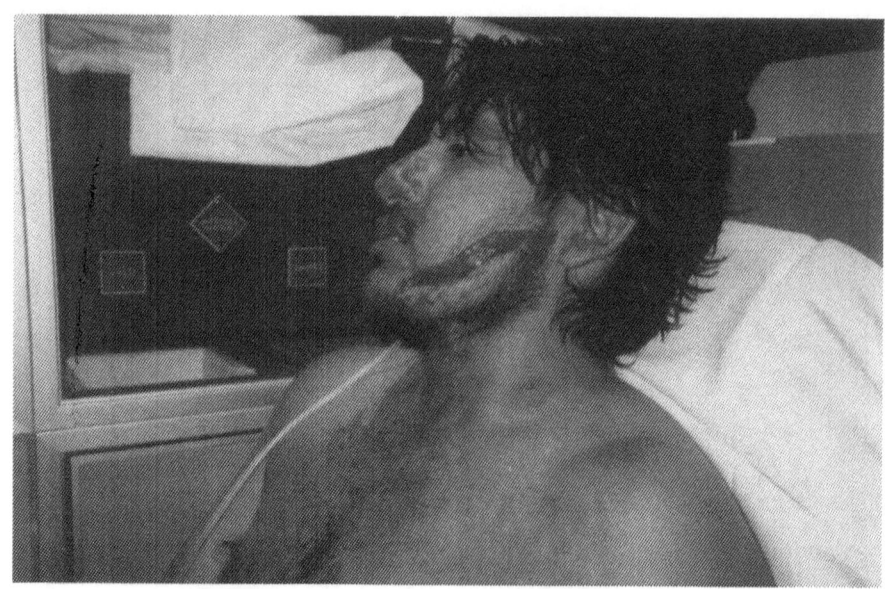

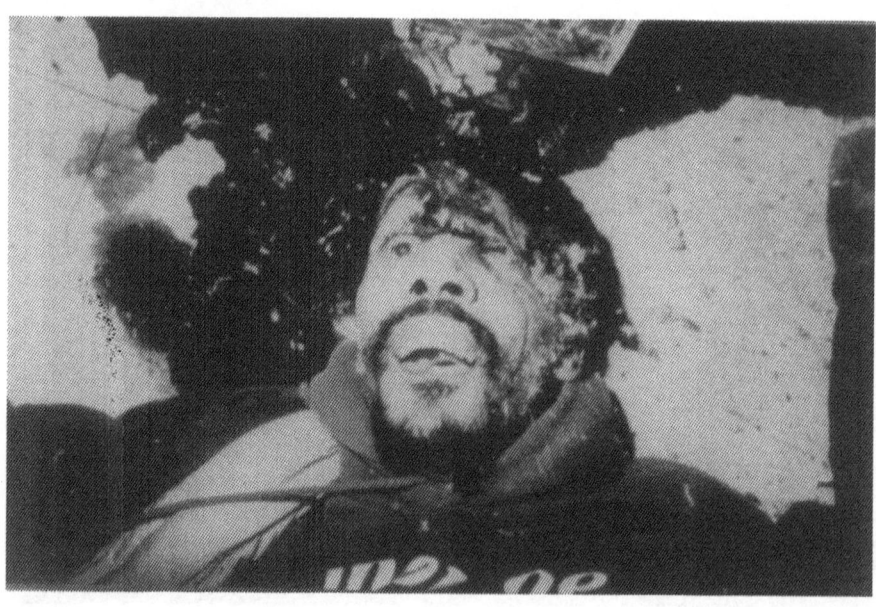

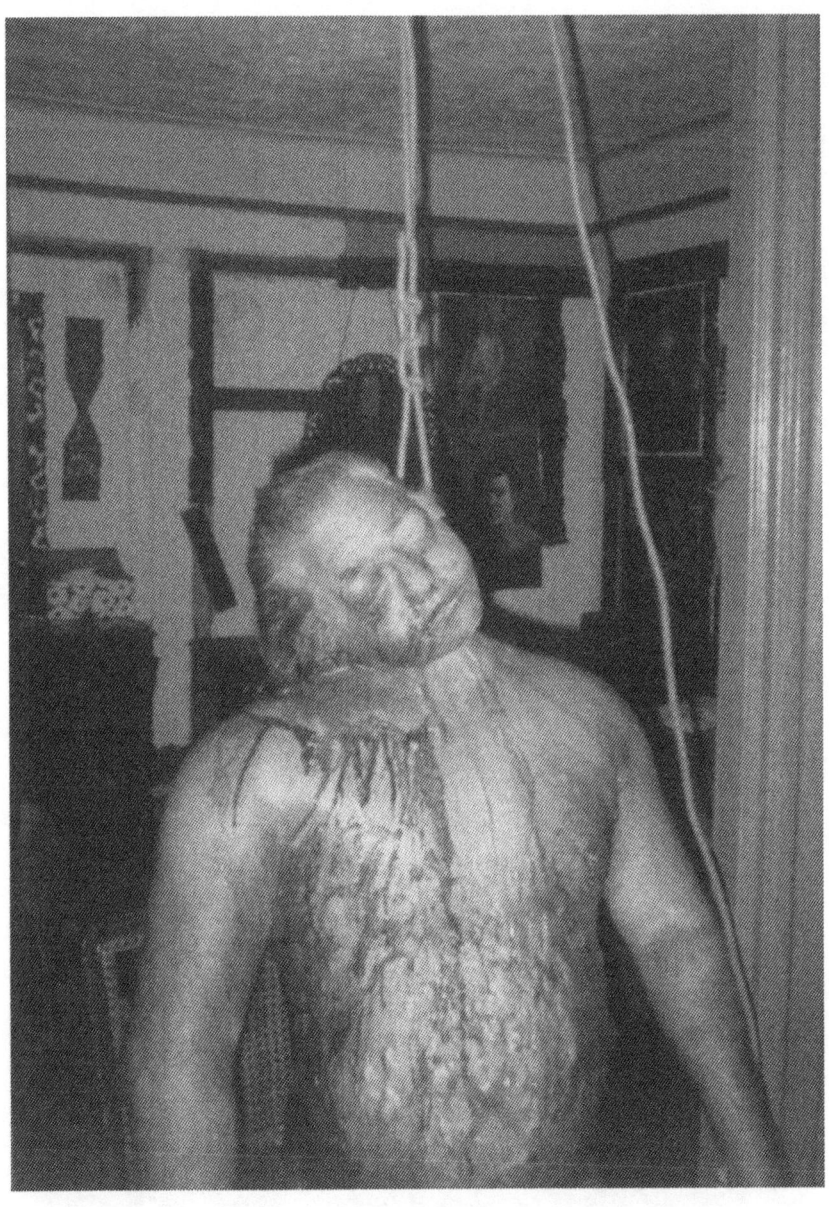

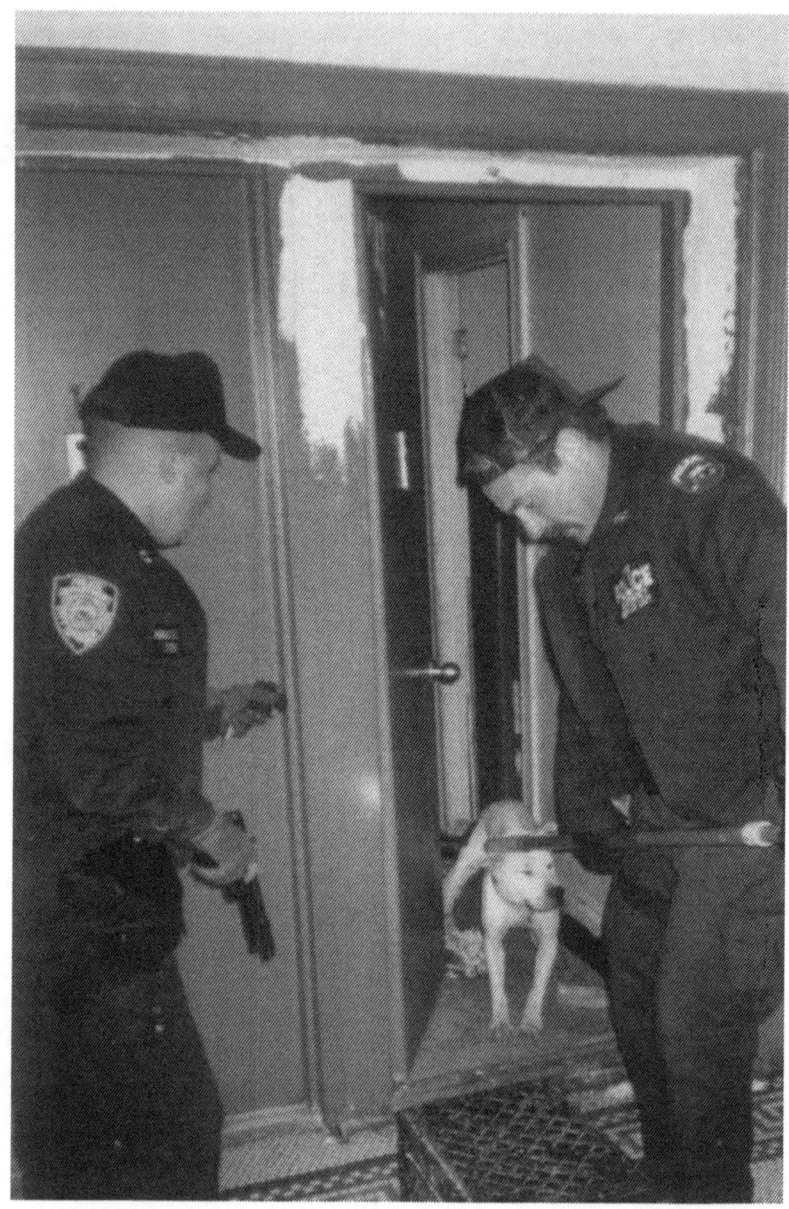

The guardian of the crackden must be removed before entering.

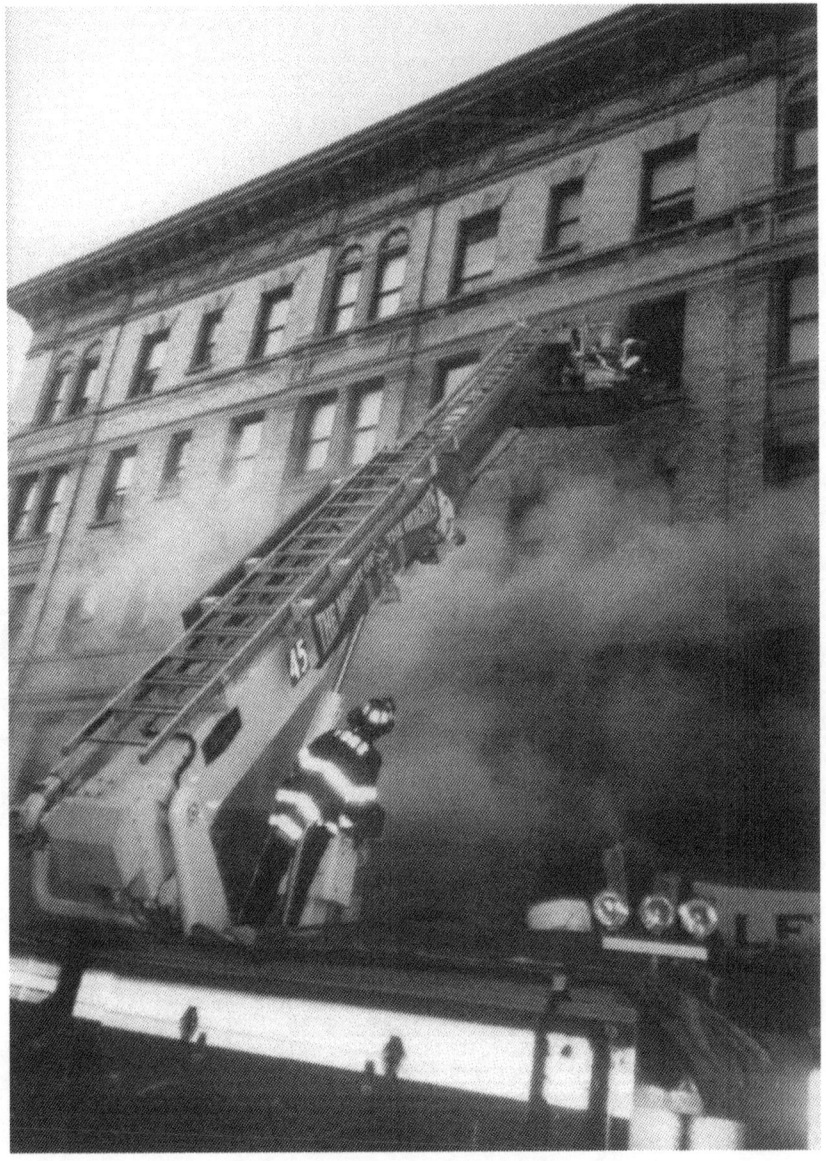

A typical fire standby.

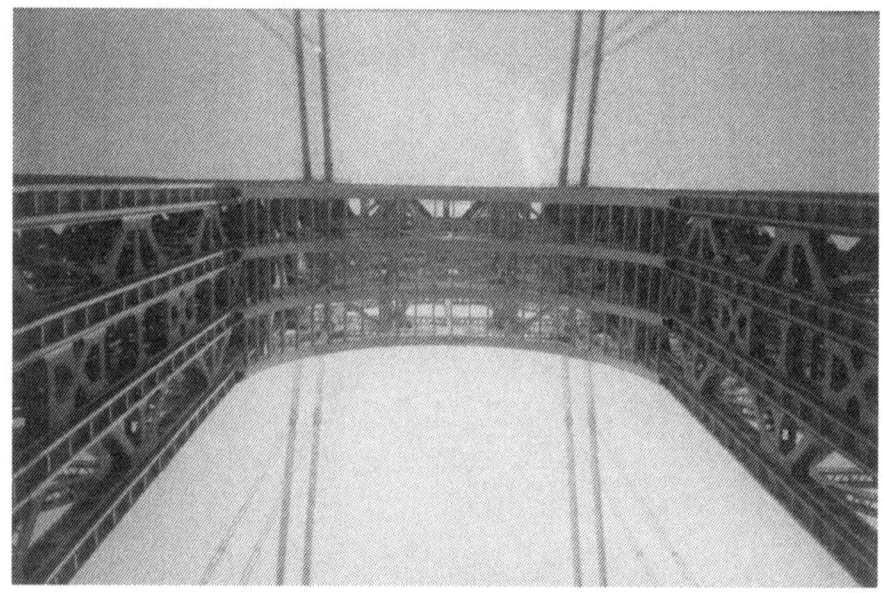

My Gateway to misery.

Chapter 10

So Christmas is coming soon. I got one more check coming before the holiday. My partners and I are getting alternate day mandates, which is hard, but I need the money having kids and all. On this day, Jason and I had decided we would come in at four o'clock, and cover the tour 3 vacancies on 18–Young. This way we would work together both tours, and just roll the unit over at midnight. Then neither one of us would be able to get mandated in the morning.

I was noticing at this time of year, you get more lonely-type people jobs. Our day started out like this, when we got called for a sick job. This elderly lady lived alone, and you could tell right away, she just needed someone to talk to. Anyway, she invited us in and told us she wasn't feeling too good, cause she wasn't eating regularly or sleeping well and she wasn't getting to see her grandchildren enough. We spoke politely, while we assessed her. We made a fuss over her, and saw that her skin and respirations were unremarkable. Her blood pressure was good, and the monitor showed a good strong sinus rhythm.

So during the flow of the conversation, I told her she had a good heart, and then I said, "see, it even looks healthy too." This made her feel good, and she asked if she could keep a piece of the strip, which I gave her about 6 inches of. We then carried her down to the rig, and brought her over to Columbia. She was quickly triaged, and sent to the waiting area, where she sat down, and struck up a conversation with a younger lady, before I was even out of there.

So we get back in service up in Washington Heights. We go available, and start to head down back to our area. We hear the radio ask 19–X-ray if they're in service yet, and they answer yes, send the job. It turns out to be a pedestrian struck, on Lenox Avenue and One–Four–Three. It's our job, but X-ray is closer, so on the way back to our corner, we stopped by their job, and saw that it was a traumatic arrest, with obvious mortal injury.

Steve and Mark were on it, and they had this guy about thirty or so. He looked really drawn from previous drug use, and was a squishy over on the northbound side of Lenox, by the park over there. He got run over by not one, not two, but three—yes three—different cars. This guy's abdomen was absolutely flat, and a lot of blood had bubbled out of his mouth, as all three cars had completely passed over him.

So I looked over him, with Jason next to me, and Mark came over to us and said, "boys, allow me to introduce you to the Lenox Avenue speed bump." We got one of those gallows humor type laughs out of that, and then went and picked up dinner at KFC, right down the block. We got to finish dinner, and about 6 o'clock, we got a job that gained me more respect for Jason, than any other job I would ever work with him.

The job was in Colonial Park houses, off the FDR Drive. It was an unconscious man, about 25 or so. The six-year-old daughter had called 911, and said her dad wasn't waking up. When we got there, she was sitting in the kitchen with the police officers, one of which was a woman, and she was being very motherly toward the little girl. The child told them, her mother and sister were shopping, and she was watching TV with her dad. He started to act different, and then laid down on the floor, and she couldn't wake him up. She tried for a long time, and then got scared, so she knew to call 911. Jason said she was right to do that, and was very smart. Anyway, we quickly assessed him as hypoglycemic. Jason explained to the girl that her father was going to be OK, and that she could help us fix him, then go to the hospital with him on our ambulance.

He takes a non-rebreather out of the oxygen bag, and explains to her that we're going to give him some fresh air, and that this will help him breathe better. I showed her the blood pressure cuff, and let her know we were going to find out how good his blood is flowing in his body. I listened to the pressure, and watched the needle on the gauge hit at 134. I told Jason he was 134/74, and he explained this was good. As I put the monitor on the patient, I thought of the little old lady we had treated previously. I got a long strip of sinus rhythm recorded, and I showed her that her dad had a good, healthy heart, and she could keep a piece of the paper that this was recorded on.

She liked this, and Jason went into the drug bag, and took out the dextrose, narcan and thiamin. Without being intimidating, or over-whelming, he gently explained this was the good medicine that was going to fix her dad. He said he was going to give him a needle, so we could get the medicine in, and he told her it wasn't going to hurt. I saw he had completely relaxed the little girl, along with the cop, whose lap she was now sitting on.

He set up an IV, and in simple, easy to understand terms, he explained what he was doing every step of the way. He started to draw up the medications. 2 mg of Narcan, 100 mg of thiamin, and as he pushes the dextrose, slowly through the IV, he told her, "he's going to wake up now." Sure enough, he came around. He was pretty fuzzy still, but his daughter's face was something that words can't describe. One of those little things, that makes your whole body tingle, as you think about destiny. Jason asked if she had any juice in the refrigerator. They did, and I took over patient care, as he, the female officer, and the little girl, went into the kitchen. They mixed up a large cup of orange juice, with a lot of sugar, and ice cubes.

As we packaged the patient, he drank all of what was in the cup. We went down to the unit, and Jason strapped the girl in on the bench, so she could sit right next to her father. He disconnected the IV, and replaced it with a saline lock, and I believe this made the kid feel better.

I took a nice slow, easy ride up to CPMC. We got her father comfortably placed in the emergency room. Before we left she gave us and the cops all, one of those hugs that would take your head off, if she was strong enough. She saved her best for Jason, and gave him a big kiss.

When we left, I told him, I thought he was a great medic, "just think, you probably affected that kids future." "Maybe some day she'll be a doctor, when she grows up." He smiled broadly, and said back to me, "yeah, or maybe a cop or a medic." I thought this is what this job is all about, and I regretted that these assignments were so few and far between. We continued to work straight through for a while, doing a few unremarkable jobs, before the next one I'm going to describe.

It was about 11:00 at night, we get a job for a cardiac arrest on a hundred and twenty-seventh street. We get met in the lobby of the building by a 10-year-old boy, who's crying, and telling us, please hurry, my mother's dead. We fly up three flights of stairs, and find a 33-year-old woman, in arrest, under the Christmas tree. There's two other kids in the room, a girl about 8 and another boy about 13. The woman's sister is also in there, and I ask her if we can get the kids out of the room. As she's stepping into the kitchen, she tells us her sister just had a seizure, she vomited, and collapsed. I start to hyperventilate, and I tell Jason, I've got one blown pupil. We notice no apparent trauma, and we're thinking she stroked during her seizure. I put her on the monitor, and I said to Jason, we have a course V-fib. Our backup arrives as I shock the woman at 200 joules, and she immediately goes asystolic.

I ask Tony if he can continue CPR, and Jimmy brings a suction unit and scoop stretcher over. Jason comes around, and drops a line in her forearm. Jimmy suctions her airway clear for me, as I send a 7.5 ET tube through her vocal cords, and begin to breathe for her. The line isn't ready yet, and as Jimmy hands an atropine and an epi to me, I tell Jason, "I'm going to drop the first load down the tube." I flush the drugs down, as Jason secures the line. He asks me to give him another epi and atropine. Tony continues CPR, and Jimmy cracks the scoop open, and readies it for our patient.

My next ten seconds are frozen in eternity, and I learned a horrible lesson the hard way. As I look up to give Jason the drugs, my eyes gaze across the Christmas tree and towards the kitchen. The little kid is looking out at us, and as our eyes made contact, my soul became scarred by her look of hopelessness. I stare like a useless bubble of goo until Tony elbows me to pass Jason the drugs. I let Jimmy ventilate the tube, and I walked over to the kitchen and asked the sister if I could use the phone to call my doctor for further orders.

By this time the patient had converted from asystole to sinus tach, but she didn't have a pulse. I informed the doctor of our situation, and he gave me an order for some IV bicarb, and a dopamine drip. We packaged the patient, and I asked the family to meet us at Harlem Hospital. On the way down the stairs, we paused on the landing to hyperventilate the patient. I whispered over to Jason, "I don't care how fucking cold-hearted it sounds, don't ever make eye-contact with a kid when you're running an arrest." He nodded and we started further down the stairs.

In the rig, we notified Harlem that we would be arriving in 3 – 4 minutes with a 33-year-old female in cardiac arrest. We got her into the ER, and they worked really hard for this patient. Ultimately, her blood pressure never came back, and she was pronounced dead about 20 minutes after we brought her in.

I really felt depressed over this job, and I was down thinking I was selfish for feeling sorry for myself. As I came out of the ER, the patient's 13-year-old son was in the lobby, and he asks me what's going on inside. For the first time in my life, I was absolutely speechless. I thought for a second, but I was blank. I felt like Ralph Kramden, when he just stands there and goes hom-ida, hom-ida, hom-ida. I looked at the kid, and I opened my mouth. It took about 3 seconds to let something out. I could only ask him, "would you like a soda or a cup of coffee?" He looked away, and nodded no. I felt like shit, that I couldn't think of anything to say to him. I really didn't envy the doctor who had to come out and talk to these kids and their aunt.

When I was back with Jason, I told him the highs and lows of this job are unimaginable. I said, "earlier I felt like we were cruising down the open road doing a hundred, now I'm asking if you can scrape me off the telephone pole."

CHAPTER 11

It's the day before Christmas Eve. Jason is off for a couple of nights, but will be back to work with me again on Christmas. I'm working with Brendan, but he's not going to be in until 1, so I got an hour to check my rig and get something to eat. I got some fried rice and an egg roll, from the Chinese restaurant on the corner. I gave the girl behind the bullet-proof plexi-glass counter $2.50, and she smiled at me and said, "Merry Christmas," as she gave me a free soda.

When Brendan came in, we signed our drugs out, and we're in service about 30 seconds, when we got a job. We weren't even to the rig yet, as Brendan had told Central that we were available from inside the station, over the portable radio. As we got to the door, they were calling us to go to One–Two–O and Lexington, for the trauma. It turns out this guy about 23 went out for a few eggnogs, after Christmas shopping. He was pretty intoxicated, and as he went into his lobby, someone followed him into the building. He got his ass kicked up on the second floor landing, during which time he got thrown down the flight of stairs and his bag of presents got robbed.

He had a nasty laceration over his eye, and a large gash on the back of his head. His left arm was broken, and his shin was severely bruised. He was slurring, and the smell of rum was obvious. We immobilized him with little resistance. His pressure and respirations were good, so I only dropped a line, and AMS'd him on the way to the hospital, after splinting his arm.

When we get in service again, we get called back down to One–Eighteen & Park for the MVA. This guy was another one who had a little too much holiday spirit. He was driving down Park Avenue, and he said his brakes failed, and that he lost control of the car. Well, he knocked down a fifty-foot metal lamppost on the corner, went through the 10-foot hurricane fence sealing off a vacant lot. He went clear across the lot, and through the other side of the gate. Steel fence was wrapped all around the front end of his car, as it landed in the basement stairwell of the building, adjacent to the lot, and crashed nose-down into the side of the structure.

The guy was fine, other than looking at a DWI charge, and I told B, "he would still be driving, if the building didn't get in his way." This got RMA'd into police custody, and we were back in service for the next victim, in no time. We headed uptown and back to our area. We parked on a hundred and fifty-eight street, and Brendan got his special of chicken wings and hot sauce. I told him I was still having agada from my fried rice, so I would have to pass on the wings, with extra grease and the death sauce. I finished up my paperwork, as Brendan chowed down.

We get a job up on One–Nine–O and Fort Washington, for an unconscious on the street. Upon arrival on the scene, we find an overdosed young Spanish male, facedown on the sidewalk, by the entrance to the "A" train.

There was some nasty heroin around at that time called homicide, and we were getting to use a lot of narcan. This guy was soaking wet from laying in a slush puddle, and he had a nice plum-shaped lump on the forehead over his eye, along with pinpoint pupils. We got him on the board, and get his clothes off on the warm rig. He was hypothermic, on top of being overdosed. We carefully wrapped him up in thick, black and gray, wool blankets. I gave him 2 mg of narcan in the bicep, as Brendan set up a line. This patient was young, but he was very shunted and constricted, and Brendan was having trouble finding a good vein. He asked me to pass him a milligram of glucagon. Then he mixed the solution, and drew up the med, as he waited for the tourniquet on the patient's arm to present any form of a vein for him.

I came around to the side and bagged the patient from the floor, between the bench and the stretcher. Brendan went to the head and sat in the captain's chair. His line was set up, and he confidently grabbed this guy's arm, and pulled his hand up next to his head, bent at the elbow. This revealed the backside of the forearm, and our favorite clutch, gotta-have-it vein, which I mentioned we called the junkie vein. We could barely see it, as B palped it like a champion, and weaved an 18 up toward the elbow. He worked hard for that line, then gave 2 more mg of narcan, the dextrose and thiamin on the way toward CPMC. I fully expected our boy to wake up, so we didn't intubate him. We were backing up to the emergency room, and B injected 2 more mg of narcan. So this guy is almost maxxed-out on narcan, by us. We gave him both glucagon IM, and dextrose IV, but he never did wake up for us. Later that night, I checked in on him, and he was on a respirator. The doctor told us he didn't know if the guy was going to recover.

We had been back in service for a little while, and we got a call for a pediatric, difficulty breathing. These jobs are usually bullshit. There's so many of them, that you can actually get beaten down by the nonsense, and be caught off-guard when something real is happening. But that didn't happen this time. It was a typical taxi job, for a paranoid 16-year-old mother. The baby was sleeping; it's after 3 in the morning, but you know, the mother is awake, and she's telling us the kid can't breathe, because he's got some congestion that you can hear. So we ask her to get the kid dressed, so we could go over to the hospital. You would think, that if you had called an ambulance, you would at least have the kid awake, if not ready. But this was OK, cause it was an easy job, and it took about 20 minutes to wake up the baby, and get him dressed. I had my paperwork finished, before we even left the apartment. We took the kid into the ER. The nurse scribbled on my ACR, and I was out of there in three minutes. I wished the nurse, and the mother a happy holiday, and I said, "I hope your baby gets better, before Christmas morning."

I then went across the street, and got a cup of coffee, and a pack of Marlboros. It was taking me like 6 cups of coffee, and 2 packs of cigarettes a night to get through my tour. I smoked in the cold, because by now, Brendan's ass was on fire from his hot wings. He was farting so bad, I had to keep the windows on the rig opened all night. And I actually asked him, if he had one of those stinky cigar stubs he could smoke.

CHAPTER 12

Christmas came and went, and I was real thankful when it was over. My personal life is in disarray from the workload, the overtime, the commuting, and the endless childcare. My daughters had a good holiday, and this assures that I'll get little sleep as the New Year arrives. The kids in the hood are off from school all week, which means they can stay up all night, as opposed to really, really late.

I'm working with Rod, a couple of nights after Christmas. He's bitching about the merger with the Fire Department that's coming up in March. He thinks we're all going to be replaced by firemen and have no jobs. I let him know that I didn't believe that to be true. I was a pretty recent hire, and they wouldn't be banging out medic classes if they were going to replace everybody. Anyway, it's a little after 2 in the morning, when the radio sends us to the Martin Luther King houses for a trauma. We get to the scene fast, and we find out there's a 12-year-old boy pinned between the roof of the elevator, and the roof of the shaft. This kid had been elevator surfing. That's when someone climbs on to the roof of the elevator from the escape hole in the elevator ceiling. Then one kid pushes the button, and the other rides on the outside of the elevator.

As the elevator approaches the shaft roof, you must then lay flat, as the space between the ceiling, and the roof of the shaft is only about 18 inches.

Well this kid is pinned in there good. It took over two hours for him to be extricated. When we arrived on the scene, he was still alive, and we could communicate with him. But by the time he was extricated, he was in traumatic arrest. He had bilateral tib/fib fractures, and both sides of his pelvis seemed to have obvious deformities. To add insult to obvious mortal injury, while the kid's hysterical parents were in the hall during the extrication process, some scumbag robbed their apartment.

When I found this out, I said to Rod, "if you believe in God and the devil, the person who did this would be in the express lane to hell." Rod's a kind of religious guy, and he took it a step further as he told me, "there was some real serious evil at work, on that scene."

So later on, we're both bummed out. Neither of us really feels like working. And when the pediatric dif breather hits at 5 o'clock in the morning, I'm feeling a lot of anger over the abuse of the system. We read the text on the KDT—vomiting child, sick, mother states child having trouble breathing. The job is all the way uptown, in those big white buildings that go over the Cross Bronx Expressway, as you approach the George Washington Bridge. So as we're heading uptown, Rod asks me to give him the callback number from the KDT. He calls the number from his cell phone, as we're riding up the FDR Drive. I hear him start talking, "good morning ma'am, this is EMS dispatch." "I'm calling to make sure everything is still all right, and to tell you the ambulance will be in front of your building in three minutes." He then asks the person, on the other end of the phone, to dress the child and meet the unit in the lobby. When we pulled up to the scene, the mother met the unit at the curb, with a three-year-old who had been experiencing mild viral symptoms for a little under a week. The vitals were very stable, and we saved the lady the five dollars that a car service ride would have cost her.

Because of Rod's quick (skell) thinking, we were able to get a much needed 20-minute caffeine, and nicotine break, as we waited for the winter sunrise. A little after 7, I'm thinking, all right, listen for a bullshit street job that we can pick up, or back-up a BLS unit on something easy, then get in for the tour change on time. As it turns out, we get sent all the way up to Vermylia Avenue, by the northern tip of Manhattan, for an inbleed.

We're both bitching about hemorrhoid jobs, and by this time I've come to realize a real inbleed might as well be an arrest, because they're so messy and there's a lot of work to be done. So of course we hike up three winding flights of stairs. We got no back-up, and the firemen looked really cool as they waved to us leaving the scene, having never even made patient contact. So we go in, and the nauseating smell of digested blood, keys me in that we're not getting off cheap with this one. The guy is laying on the floor of the bathroom, soaked in smelly, dark, coffee-grind blood. There's a large amount soaked through his pajamas, forming a puddle on the pink-and-white, small tiled floor. The guy is real lethargic, and I tell Rod, "I'll get a BP," as he puts a non-rebreather mask on the man's face, and pumps up the oxygen. We know what's coming with the pallor, and poor skin turgor. I can hear a thready pulse of about 150, as I get a blood pressure of seventy over forty.

Rod tells me he'll go get the scoop stretcher, while I hit the lines. I straddle this man's bloody body, and as I kneeled towards the torso, I said to Rod, "I love my kids, that's why I'm here." "What's your excuse?" Rod just shook his head as he walked out.

I hit a 14-gauge IV, in the left forearm, then another in the right. I ran them wide open, and was securing the second line in place, as Rod came back in. He looked really wiped-out, and we both knew the real work hadn't even started yet. This guy was large, about 6'3" and over 240 pounds. After cutting his drenched pajamas off of him, we got him packaged, and asked Central to give a notice to the Allen Pavilion, that we were coming.

We had a hard time just winding around the bathroom, and out of the apartment. By the time we got out into the hallway, I was already soaked with sweat. We got down one landing, and rested about 10 seconds, before we had to lift the scoop upright, to make a turn. We got down to the second floor, and my arms were getting numb. I could see Rod was feeling weak also. We put him on the ground for a second, then we decided we would rest the stretcher on the steel ball of the banister post, at the next landing. This would allow us to pivot, and continue down to the next floor, without awkward and strenuous lifting and turning. Well the scoop stretcher has some wide gaps in between the sidebars, and the aluminum slats. As we made the pivot, the stretcher slid sideways, about six inches, and the top of the post got stuck in between the stretcher bar and the slat. "This sucks," I said. I could see by Rod's face, he was ready to quit. I told him, "there's no way to explain this, no one coming to help us, we gotta get this done." He looked at me, while I was struggling to keep the stretcher from tipping sideways, and dumping our patient. I told him, "my arms are numb, we got one shot." "On three, lift up hard." We counted together—One – Two – Three, and we both thrust upward with everything we had left. The stretcher popped up over the post ball, with a loud snapping noise. We bent the slat, but we got it over the handrail, and slid it slowly down the last five steps.

On the last landing, we slid the scoop down the steps, smoothly and slowly, like a sled. When we got it to the lobby, I could barely lift the patient off the floor, onto the vehicle stretcher. It was still real cold, so we had to get him on the bus quickly, and somehow, we did.

When this job was finally completed, I thought that my burnt bodega coffee never tasted better, as I used it to put down a jelly donut, that I think the New York Rangers used that night for their hockey puck.

We returned to the station, and when I got to the parking lot, my car wouldn't start. I thought this only happens on nights like this. I went back to the station, and found out I could do four hours overtime, on a BLS unit. I figured I'm already trashed, but at least this will pay for the new car battery I need to get. Being back on a unit allowed me to get over to the auto parts store, and get shook down. In between bullshit taxi jobs, I was able to get the new battery installed. I turned the car over, and when my overtime was done, I headed home.

I was so tired, I was seeing purple dots out of the side of my eyes. As I got off the Brooklyn Bridge I dazed out for a second, and I crashed my car into the raised curb on the exit ramp. I got a flat, bent my rim, and broke my tie rod. I was so fucking pissed, I was spitting stomach acid. I needed to get towed, and with the repair, it cost me $220. I called the station, and Jimmy answered the phone, "Station 18, desk lieutenant, how can I help you?" I told Jimmy that I still wasn't home. I was raving about being so tired I crashed my car. I waited for him to tell me to take a night off and rest. After making sure I was still all right, he said, "Daniel, you're a big boy. Go get some rest, and I'll see you in the morning." I stared at the phone in disbelief as my quarter ran out. I slammed the phone down so hard I fucked up my wrist. When I finally got home, it was after 6 o'clock. I fell asleep in my uniform, and slept for about three hours. I ate a cold sandwich, as I warmed up my piece-of-shit of a car. I cursed it out, and went back to work, unbathed, and in the same smelly uniform I had worn the night before to start the whole fucking endless process again.

CHAPTER 13

New Year's eve was a mulage of intoxicated, puking madmen, with a few overdoses and MVA's thrown in. I worked with Brendan, and we were both pretty irritable. I remember getting an OD, in a hallway, by Mt. Morris Park. This guy was in the lobby, covered in vomit, with typical pinpoint pupils. Well we walk in, and Brendan takes two bristojets of narcan, and pushes one in each of this guy's arms, right through his jacket, shirt, and whatever else he was wearing. Anyway, he gives this guy about two and a half minutes, before he starts shaking him, and says, "get the fuck up Hector, come on let's go." So this guy starts waking up, and he's acting like he was just sleeping. Brendan stays in action, and he tells the guy, "shut up asshole, we know you've been doing dope, and you probably still got some on you, don't you." The guy is acting scared, and B says to him, "get the fuck outta here, before the cops come, or else you're getting arrested." As our junkie is leaving, he also tells him, "don't let me find you again tonight, or I'll just drop you off at the Two–Six precinct." So the guy wanders off, and Brendan tells Central we got a 90 (no patient). Then we headed up to One–Ten and Broadway for some bagels and coffee.

We get a job for a "sick" passenger in the subway, on a Hundred and Thirty-fifth and St. Nick. We go down into the tombs, and a train is stopped in the station. There's a minefield of vomit on the platform, as we're led down to the end, by the cops. We enter the last car of the train, and we see a guy, slumped in the corner seat, and he looks like he's sleeping. As we approach, I tell Brendan, "another two stops, and he would have been X-ray's problem." We get a little closer, and I notice he's a good shade of purplish-gray around his head, and he's stinking. Brendan pokes him, and this guy is completely stiff. I say to the cops, "he's probably been dead since Brooklyn." We make him an 83, and leave the body with PD, to be removed by BLS, which was now arriving.

The night continued into morning, and when I left to return home, it was snowing.

So I come to work on my birthday. I haven't told anyone what day it is, and I'm pretty bummed out, because no one remembered. I'm working with Jason tonight, but he's going to be late. So I'm talking with Sy, as I'm checking out my rig. I haven't seen him in a while, which is strange. When I ask how he's been, he tells me he was in the hospital the last few days, with pneumonia. But now he is feeling better, and when he gets medical clearance, is going back on the rig.

He notices that I'm feeling depressed, and pushes the issue, asking me why I ain't myself tonight. I try to blow it off, but when he asks, "what's the matter, did you and Jason have a falling out?" I said "no." I told him I had just got done working the holidays for the fourth year in a row, and I didn't even get a card for my birthday. He told me he could understand, and I remember in November, when he told me his birthday sucked, and nobody remembered it. So I said, "see, we got something in common." We smoked a couple of cigarettes, and I heard 19–Victor get assigned to an arrest in my area. It sounded like a job we would eat up, but we wouldn't be in service for a half-hour.

When Jason gets in, we quickly get in service and pick up a job for a MVA on One–Two–Five and Two. A BLS unit is responding from St. Luke's, we're coming from the station on One–Three–Six and Lenox. So we get there a little ahead of them. When we get on the scene, we find two young females in a car that has sustained very serious front-end damage, from a head-on collision with a van. The driver of the van had minor injuries, and RMA'd, but the two girls in the car were really busted up good. The girl behind the wheel was a diabetic, and went hypoglycemic prior to the accident, while driving. Her head hit the steering wheel, and she was literally scalped, as if by Indians in a cheap movie. Her hair was pushed back to the center of her head, and a few inches of her skull was clearly visible.

Her friend smashed her head into the windshield, causing it to break like a spider web with red trails. Her hair was stuck in the broken weave of glass, and I had to cut it before we could remove her. Me and Jason split up with the BLS crew. He takes the trauma bag and our spare restock bag on the BLS bus. I get an EMT to drive our rig, and we both work immobilized patients on the fly en route to Harlem Hospital.

After the job we do a quick restock, and start our night with a proper breakfast of fried rice and chicken wings. I come out with the food, and some crack head is asking me for a quarter. I tell him no and I move on, as I'm thinking, it's almost three in the morning, and this guys probably making more than me grubbing change on Lenox Avenue.

The night turns into morning and we're bombarded with the usual assault of asthmatics, drunks and dif breathers. As the sun rises, we find out we're both getting mandated, so I tell myself, Happy Birthday, did you expect anything different? We roll the unit over in the morning, and we get a job for a cardiac arrest. It's in one of these really skeevy, roach-infested, single room occupancy motels, on Park Avenue, next to the Metro North ell.

We get on the scene and this guy is sprawled half on the bed with his head and upper torso hanging off the edge. He's been in this garbage filled room so long, that the cats that were stuck in the room with him ate his eyes, and his whole body was a blackish-purple. By now the cops were here and they were asking us if it looked suspicious. I said, "I really can't tell, but by the looks of the syringe on the table, and the numerous crack vials, and empty liquor bottles around the room, it was probably an overdose." I then looked at Jason, and said, "looks yummy, doesn't it," as I picked maggot off the head of our corpse. I told the cops he was all theirs, and I left the room with things sticking to my feet. So I purposely walked through a puddle before I got back on the rig to let Central know we had an 83 left with PD.

By now the world is in full swing, as I say to Jason, "it's bad luck to give the vampire crew jobs in the sunlight." And he asks me, "bad luck for us, or the patients?" So we get sent into the projects on fifth avenue, and a hundred and Thirty-fifth Street, literally across the street from the hospital.

Basically this woman has really bad menstrual cramps, but doesn't want to cross the street and go to Harlem. She wants us to taxi her down into the barrio, to Mt. Sinai. She's a real asshole, and we can't even begin to speak intelligently with her. I'm bitching about people taking advantage of the system with this sort of nonsense, and she snaps at me, "you all are just a bunch of stupid motherfuckers, you gots to take me to the hospital." So I'm thinking, this is original, I haven't been called a stupid motherfucker in about three hours, as I say to her, "you're clearly telling me you have bad cramps from your period." "I'll take you across the street, if you need to go to the hospital." Well that did it. She's getting all political now, and me and Jason are a bunch of racist motherfuckers, cause we don't want to taxi her to Mt. Sinai.

So enough is enough. We finally give in, and I ask her to come down to the rig, cause her chauffeur is waiting. It's a quiet ride down the vertical urinal. When we get to the rig, we put out the step stool for her to use to climb in. As she does, she cackles to me, "you all would treat me better if I was white." I didn't miss a step. I responded, "no, I would treat you like a white idiot," and then proceeded to have my unit out of service, for over an hour, on one of the purest forms of bullshit jobs you could ever receive.

So we leave the hospital, and Jason gets us some nuclear Spanish coffee, that's making the little hairs on the back of my neck stand up. We head back uptown, towards our area, and I'm thinking the day will soon be over. Then I can go home for a change of pace, and a different form of aggravation.

Anyway, we get one more job that morning, another classically intelligent person. The radio bellows, "One–Four–Three and Lenox for the burn." We respond that we're sixty-three, en route. We go through yet another, piss-filled elevator, and leave our wet footprints down the hall. We get to the apartment as we find a woman, whose head looks like a burnt match. Like I said, she's a real genius. She was dying her hair, the color all these old ladies use that makes it look blue. Anyway, she decided to light a cigarette while doing this and POOF. Well, she has no eyebrows or eyelashes, and a lot of her hair was singed off to the scalp, causing a terrible smell. She had huge blisters on her face and head, which were proliferated by this gop, that she had smeared all over them. She was in pain, but her airway was in no danger, so she could easily explain to us what happened. Apparently after she torched herself, she smeared something called beewax all over the burns. I fathomed this wasn't helping much, and we took her over to Harlem hospital.

When the job was completed, I was outside the emergency room, and me and Jason started laughing at the concept of her spontaneously combusting while dying her hair. We went out of service, overtime personnel, and as we walked over to the parking lot together, Jason said, "I hope she gets a wig soon." I responded that I didn't think she would be allowed out in public without one, and that her hair would grow back in about a year and a half.

I was happy to leave, and I smoked a fat joint on the way home, and occasionally still laughed about our last job. I paid the legal extortion to go over my seven-dollar bridge, and was finally home, almost two hours after I left the station.

CHAPTER 14

It's a brutally cold night, and me and Brendan are in service, as we're talking about our merger with FDNY. He's telling me it's a hostile takeover, not a merger. After all, the city isn't burning down like it used to due to better building codes, and so forth. You don't have whole blocks going up anymore. So what do you do? The other thing is the fire department has been predominately white Irish males for over a hundred and fifty years. They had been ordered to integrate a few years ago by the government, and had been found to be non-compliant. So what's the answer? Make firemen certified first responders and then absorb EMS, the ultimate equal opportunity employer.

So as it goes down, we appropriately enough, join the fire department on St. Patrick's day. We were considered civilian employees of FDNY. While even Sanitation, is considered a uniformed service, with all the benefits that go with that. We had to live by the same bullshit rules as EMS, while trying to uphold a higher standard. The fire department gained 3,500 new employees as part of FDNY bureau of EMS, a completely different entity than the actual firefighters. They became integrated on paper, while the core essentially remained unchanged. They get a bigger government budget, and a big pay raise, because allegedly now they're doing their jobs and ours. If the public knew how fucked up things really were, they'd be scared. And we remained, I believe, the only fire department in the country, where you get promoted from paramedic to fireman, a very backward form of thinking.

Our unit designations have changed, but our areas are still the same. The BLS units are A's followed by a number. The paramedic units are

M's followed by a number. For example, 18–Young became medic–166 or M166. 11–Frank became ambulance–162 or A162.

This was very confusing to most people, and it just didn't sound right. It didn't last long, and for whatever reason, the unit designations went back to the old system. So as far as the medic rigs went, the designations went as follows, 18–Young became 16–Victor; 19–X-ray became 13–Willy, and 19–Victor became 13–X-ray. This is how I'll refer to the units the rest of the way.

I've been working with Brendan on 13–Willy the past few nights, and like said before the cold was ball-biting. We got a job for a fire standby, which really sucked. An abandoned building was burning up good. About 4 of the 6 floors were involved and we were out there about three hours. When the fire was out, the building looked really cool, because all the water was freezing over and making thousands of icicles along the whole building front and side. But the best thing was that there were no patients to be treated or transported.

About a half-hour after sunrise, we get called for a cardiac arrest on One–Six–Six and Riverside, on a park bench. As we get to the scene, I know this is from the homeless shelter two blocks away. Brendan lights a cigar and walks over to this guy, whose half sitting, half laying, on his side, with a bottle of Wild Turkey bourbon next to him. It was a big liter bottle, and there were only about two shots left in it. Anyway, he's frozen stiff and gray. I look over at B and I ask, "excuse me sir, what flavor of bumsicle can I get for you this morning?"

We left our 83 with PD, to be removed from the scene by BLS. This guy was so rigamortised and frozen, they had to transport him down to the morgue sitting on the stretcher.

At the end of our tour, I figured I could pick up some easy overtime on a BLS unit for four hours. I cut a deal with Jimmy, so that by volunteering for the OT, I would go to the bottom of the mandate list, which would save me for all of about two days.

So it's a good morning. I'm three hours in and we only did one job, a nonsense abdominal pain that we banged out with no problem. We get a call at the park on One–Four–O and Lenox for an injury. The text states male caller, at the scene, can't walk. So I'm thinking this is easy bullshit, right near the hospital, then I'm done. I know it's not Levi, because it didn't come over as a seizure. So we get led over to a stoop on a hundred and fortieth street, and I ask this guy, "what's the matter today sir?" And he tells me, "doc, you gotta sew the flesh back on my legs." I said, "excuse me," and he repeated himself, adding the meat on his legs was falling off. I carried him over to the vehicle with Mel, my EMT partner. When we cut his pants off, we had found that this patient had tied newspaper around his legs, under his pants, to try to stay warm. Well that was four days ago. By now the paper was soaked wet, and the string had impaired his circulation below his knees. The rope had cut through his flesh, down to the bone, and yes, his necrosed flesh was hanging off the bone. There really wasn't a thing we could do, other than comfort measures.

We transported him to Harlem hospital, where his legs had to be amputated, and he was letter discharged to a nursing home. I felt bad that people had to live like this, and it bothered me that something terrible had to happen to someone before they could get help.

CHAPTER 15

The weather will be turning soon, and with the warmer climate will come an increase in call volume. I've been hanging out with a lot of the guys that work tour three, which seems to be where most of the party people work. I'm getting to know a lot of the guys that are on these units, so I've been coming in early to cover overtime on the evenings. Then I can't get mandated for the following morning.

On this particular afternoon, I'm working with Mark. He's a really good guy. We get along great, and work real well together. I'm in service on 16–Victor, which I let Mark use on the evenings, but it's my stage on overnights.

I know it's been busy lately, and this day is no different. Right before dinner, we get hit for a confirmed double shooting, by 3333 Broadway. This is a real busy area, and a lot of trauma goes on over there. Basically you have about thirty thousand people living on a quarter square mile of modern hi-rises. Anyway, we get on the scene, and there's already a big crowd, and a lot of cops. Sy and Manny are backing us up on 11–Frank. This is their area and they arrive quickly. We see where the crime scene starts. We got one guy around thirty-five, he's shot in the ear, and the exit wound is out his eye, on the opposite side. His eye is dangling down the side of his face, about two inches from where the slug tore its way out of his head. He's laying between two parked cars, on the curb, and there's a lot of blood pooling up in the gutter.

We got another guy about the same age, only skinnier, laying on the sidewalk, shot in the back of the head and out his mouth. This guy is a

DOA also. Well, me and Mark are talking to Sy, on the other side of where Manny is. So Manny starts walking over to us and goes real close to the bodies, and takes a good hard look at these guys. As he starts walking out again, you hear this cop yell out, "hey OJ, can you stop leaving bloody footprints in my crime scene?" As it turns out, Manny walked right through a large puddle of blood and really disrupted things. So he's really embarrassed, and I guess the brains on the sidewalk must have shaken him up.

So we're making fun of him, and he's very humble, as he says, "I'm just going to crawl on over here and do my paperwork." He puts his ACR on the hood of the car, and starts writing, as the same cop walks up to him and taps him on the back, and says "thanks a lot, I think there were fingerprints left on the hood of the car." "Whoever did this is going to send you a Christmas card."

Well I thought Manny was going to drop dead over there. He slinked back to his unit holding his head low. The cop told Sy, "you should take him back to the station, and let him start his tour over like it's a new day." He apologized, and said, "Manny's really a good guy. He was probably just shook." But we never let him live it down, and he was forever known as Manny-crime-scene from that day on.

So, after doing a taxi job up to CPMC, we get a call for a cardiac arrest on One–Three–Eight and Powell. 11–Frank is again on our back, and I say to Sy over the air, the text on the KDT states it's an infant. They get on the scene first, and we hear Sy asking over the radio, "16–Victor…ETA, ETA." I tell him we're less than thirty seconds out, as Mark's got us flying down Seventh Avenue. Sy says he's jetting, as we pull up to the building. He and Manny-crime-scene come running out.

Sy's got the oxygen bag strapped over his shoulder, and he's got the kid cradled in one big arm, with his bicep supporting the head. He's getting the kid hyperventilated, and rushing towards my rig. Mark jumped in the back with me, and Manny got behind the wheel, leaving the BLS vehicle on the scene. Mark and Sy put the kid on our short board, as the rig took off toward Harlem Hospital.

Sy told us the baby was twenty-eight days old. His mother put him in the cradle about 7:00, and when she checked him at 7:20, he wasn't breathing, and was blue. Mark continued to bag the baby, and Sy did rapid CPR with the tips of two fingers. I set a 3.0 ET tube, on the fly, and went in with the smallest straight blade. I pushed the tube in between the tiny vocal cords, and I thought to myself, stay focused, stay in control.

Mark confirmed the tube was good, as I held this baby's life between my fingers. As we pulled back into the ambulance bay at Harlem Hospital, I told Sy we had a brachial pulse, and the monitor was banging out a strip of sinus tach at 160. I continued to breathe for the infant, and cradled him like a football with my right arm, and held the tube with my left hand. Mark bagged for me, and we quickly walked simultaneously into the pediatric emergency room, with our post-arrest infant.

Because we got the baby back, we found out a couple of days later that he had been diagnosed with whooping cough, and would wind up getting better and being discharged. I was told that if he hadn't been resuscitated, he would have gone into the statistics as a SIDS baby. This was one of my most rewarding jobs, and I still tell myself that was my personal Super Bowl. Win or lose, on instincts. These types of jobs always hit when you least expect it. Things happen so fast, it's almost surreal, when I reflect back on it.

After the baby job, I still had half a tour left with Mark, then I was going to roll over and work with Jason all night. I was starting to feel real productive, when Levi flagged us down at about 8:15. I was happy to see him, as we told Central we were flagged at One–Four–O and Lenox, for a seizure. We spent about 10 minutes talking to him. He grubbed a cigarette and a quarter off me. When we got in the back of the rig, I called Central to let them know we were en route to hospital 07. Then I held the radio out toward Levi, and keyed it up. He slurred, "this is Levi, I'm going to hospital 07—that's Harlem." My lieutenant didn't think this was too funny, but he knew we were just feeling good. And we talked more about the double shooting, and the infant resuscitation than we did about Levi's unauthorized transmission.

After Levi, we took a break on an available status. A lot of people we work with were asking us about the baby job we had done. And all four of us were getting a lot of congratulations. For the first time in a while, I was looking forward to my next tour. An hour after Levi, we got an unconscious heroine overdose on One–Four–Seven and Douglas. I was thinking that I even like these jobs tonight. I hit a line and gave our famous coma cocktail of dextrose, narcan and thiamin. And, about two minutes later our patient woke up, and was actually grateful to us. He said he didn't intend to fall out in the street, as I whispered to Mark, "not too many people do." We then took the shuttle ride back to Harlem Hospital.

Mark was getting off soon, and I would take over the unit with Jason. I guess he ran into someone in the parking lot, that told him it was busy, because when I saw him in the station, he already knew about the double shooting we were on earlier, and he congratulated us on getting the baby back.

Jason was excited, as he asked if I still had anything left to work with him. I responded, "come on, your talking to me, remember." The good thing was, I had taken care of the unit all day, and the bus was fully stocked and ready to go. 16–Victor was in service, on tour 1, before Mark was even out the door.

It's about two minutes after midnight, and we're getting a job over on One–Four–Six and Douglas for a trauma. As I'm driving over to the job, I say to Jason that I was just here a few minutes ago doing an overdose. As this turns out, a cop is there, and he's got this guy who put his hand through a plate glass window. There's about a quart of blood running down the sidewalk, along the curb. The cops got a handkerchief wrapped around his wrist, and he tells us when he pulled up the man was gushing blood. He says, "watch this," as he takes the handkerchief off, and blood spurts out from this patient's wrist, arching about four feet. I said "OK, I believe you, let's get some pressure on that." We carried this guy over to the rig, and he's telling me he's dizzy, as we lay him down on the stretcher. We give him some oxygen, and I drop a fourteen in him, and start squeezing the fluid in. I'm trying to calm him down, so we can help him, as Jason tells me his blood pressure is 76/40.

He started driving, and asked dispatch to let the hospital know we were coming. En route, I dropped a 16 gauge IV in his wounded arm, and started to run another 1000 bag. When we got out of the ER, Jason slapped me on the back, and said "good job, Dano." "That was life saving trauma." I felt real good, because until that moment, I hadn't even realized this. I said, "thanks, I'm on a roll tonight." Jason told me it sounded more like I was in the zone, and that he wanted me in the back of the rig all night. I told him this was fine with me, and I knew we would continue to kick ass, all night long.

I realized I hadn't eaten all day, and we tried to get something on One–Two–Five and Amsterdam. As I watched my cheeseburger sizzle, we got a job for an unconscious at 30 Hamilton Place. This wasn't too far away. It's one of those single-room occupancy welfare hotels, and there's a lot of drugs and violence over there.

We get to the scene, and a Spanish woman about twenty-five, tells us her friend won't wake up, and is snoring loudly. I'm thinking this is going to be worthy of an incredible bullshit award. But when we get in, we find another young Spanish woman, out-cold on the bed. She's got a huge purple lump on her forehead, and one of her pupils is dilated.

Me and Jason don't even need to talk, we know she's fucked, and we know what we gotta do. I ask the friend, "how did she get that lump on her head," and she told me the girls boyfriend punched her this morning. The patient took an oral airway, and I started to hyperventilate her. Jason put the monitor on, and did a blood pressure. I'm thinking, I don't care if Mike Tyson hit her, one punch wasn't going to do this. So her blood pressure is 220/120 and her heart rate is 40. Jason sets a line, and I easily drop a 7.5 tube in her. We have some discussion as to what protocols to run, as we both agree we have a bleed inside the head. We got her packaged, and took a straight run down to St. Luke's. I continued to hyperventilate her, and was thankful that at least she wasn't having any seizures.

I found out a few days later, that she never did wake up. Her boyfriend had been arrested and charged with murder. He had conked her with a full beer bottle, and I had kind of expected to hear something stupid like that. Anyway, we went back to One–Two–Five and Amsterdam, after the job, and I paid $4 for a dry, cold cheeseburger, and soggy French fries, which had waited over an hour for me.

So we're back at the station, in service. I'm trying to do a restock, while I inhale my meal. I'm talking with Sy, who's still hanging around, and Derrick and Ziffy. Zif tells us that me and Jason are getting a big time rep as a kick-ass unit. I responded to him that we fear no job. We'll back up any unit, anywhere, anytime, no problem. And he said, "I see that." I continued my restock. I told Sy if he was still here in the morning, I would treat him to breakfast. Then we headed up to the triangle on One–Three–Six and St. Nick, to watch the traffic drive by.

As expected, we didn't get to idle too long and we got sent down to One–Eleven and Riverside Drive, for the asthmatic on the street. I said to Jason "I know who this is," and he told me he did too. We figured, OK, we'll relax on this one for a little while. And when we told Central we were responding, 11–Zebra went available from the ER, and said this was their job, and they would pick it up for us. I thought this was really cool for them to do this, and it showed respect.

So we decide to cruise around the neighborhood for a little while, and as we go by One–Four–O and Lenox, I could see Levi has already been discharged, and is back drinking in his living room, which is his favorite park bench.

It was getting late, and I was starting to feel the effect that the day was having on my body. I told Jason that my back was really hurting. I didn't feel like I was working really hard or anything, it's just a constant fatigue.

We get a job on One–Three–Seven, off Broadway, for a shot. We hear it go over PD, so we're on it before Central even calls us. As the radio summons, "16–Victor, 16–David…One–Three–Seven and Broadway for the shot," we're less than a minute out. I say to Jason, "this is right where we did the double just eight hours ago, and this has reprisals written all over it."

This one was in a third floor apartment, in a smaller building across from the complex. We get this guy, who's about twenty-five. He's shot once in the back of the head, with no exit wound. It's a huge hole, oozing thick blood, and the back of his head feels like slush. Unfortunately, the bullet left his medulla in place, thus leaving him with a carotid pulse and agonal respirations. Ziffy and Derrick backed us up, and the four of us got him on a board. I held his head together with a multi-trauma bandage, as Zif slid a collar on him. Jason set up two trauma lines, and hit one, as I attempted to intubate this guy. There was a lot of blood coming up this patient's airway, and I couldn't get a good look down at the vocal cords. I aimed high, and I dropped the tube in. I listened for lung sounds, but found out my tube was a belly-bomb.

I extubated him, as Jason hit a second line. I tried to get another look, to no avail. I said I'll do it down in the rig, and Jason knew I would, as he suggested that we get the fuck off the scene. And the four of us humped the long-board down the stairs.

It was hard to keep this guy's head together, and we were trailing blood all the way out. I set up a smaller 7.0 tube, and J suctioned the airway for me. We took off towards St. Luke's with Derrick driving one rig, and Zif driving the other. We got about 60 cc's of blood out of the patient's mouth, and I saw the vocal cords for like a tenth of a second, before the blood outflowed the suction. They were high, and a little off-center, to the right. I couldn't hyperextend this guy, so I aimed high again, and pushed the tube in where I had seen the white lines of the airway entrance. The tube was good, and we continued to work.

When we got into the emergency room, I noticed dark, army-green brain matter on my stretcher. We stuck around, until the patient was pronounced dead, then went back to the station, for extensive decontamination.

Sy was still there, and he was kind of high, cause the tour three, after work cocktail party was in full effect. He came over to me, and asked "was that shooting good?" I responded, "hell yeah, look some of his brains are still here." He started laughing as he grabbed the hose and started spraying down the floor of the rig. Then he went back in his memory, and was telling me a whole bunch of the back-in-the-day stories, until Lt. Lardass came and told us she had put us back in service.

We only got one more job that morning, and we were 87'd by BLS, so we could get off on time. This was good for me, because I was on sixteen hours, and I felt like I had just worked like a $5 whore.

It didn't matter to Jason though, because he got mandated, and had to stay six more hours. When I was leaving, I woke up Sy from sleeping on the station bench, and asked him if he wanted to eat. We drove down to One–Three–Two and Lenox, where for $4, you can get eggs, sausage, corned beef hash, bacon, grits, toast, coffee and orange juice. We ate so much, that we needed to be rolled out of the place.

I drove home thinking I had a fantastic night. When I opened my glove compartment to get change, I noticed a well-deserved fatty of a bone, I had forgotten about. So I slipped in my Steely Dan tape, and lit up. I thought for once the EMS god had chosen to smile on me, instead of lifting his leg. I got a decent amount of sleep, and I played with my kids a little that afternoon. Then went back that night to start the whole fucking endless process over again.

CHAPTER 16

I'm working with Jason tonight in good spring weather. Things have been going really well, and we have established ourselves as a kick-ass, frontline unit, that students are even starting to seek out. The night started out with a cardiac arrest. It turns out the neighbors of this old lady hadn't seen her since the end of January, so they decided she must be dead in her apartment, and called 911. Well, by the smell coming out, we thought they just might be right. So I'm thinking, hmmm, no one's seen or cared for her in a couple of months, but suddenly in the middle of the night, they think something may be wrong. I couldn't help myself. I had to ask, "what changed in the last three and a half months, that you thought to call an ambulance tonight?"—Anyway, a visitor to the building told her friend, it smelled like death by that door. Then it suddenly occurred to her, that she hadn't seen her neighbor in a while. So no one's answering the telephone or the bell. ESU comes, and pops the door. Well sure enough, this woman is up against it, dead.

We could only get the door open a crack. As I shine my maglight into the apartment, I see garbage stacked from the floor to the ceiling, taking up three-quarters of the room. We push the door in as far as we can, and when we enter we see this naked, three hundred pound woman, lying in a pile of old newspaper, shoes and clothes, and a lot of useless items in brown paper bags. There are cockroaches clearly visible everywhere, and it looks like an explosion in a poor box, around her body.

The neighbor asks from out in the hall, "how come it smells so bad in there," and "is she dead?" I looked over at the body, and saw it was covered in green mold. I thought she resembled Swamp Thing. Her mouth was bright red, and starting to skeletize, where the rats had started to eat the soft tissue around it. So I replied, "yeah, I think so," as I lit a big smelly cigar, and puffed away.

We stepped out of the apartment, back into the hall, and this woman is screaming and crying hysterically. When we left the building, Jason says to me, "I don't want to sound insensitive, but how much could that neighbor have cared, that she waited so long to even think of knocking on her door, but then she gets all emotional, when she finds out the woman is dead?"

We went into service, as we told Central we had an 83 left with PD, and headed over to our area. We get a job down in the barrio, for an unconscious female, on Paladino, off of one sixteen. An older guy who had been walking his dog leads us behind the school on that block. In the back corner of the schoolyard, up against the building, there's a Spanish woman, about twenty, who had been raped. Her face was busted up really bad, and her pants and underwear were still down below her knees. She was kind of lethargic, and had pinpoint pupils.

We carefully and gently wrapped her in a white sheet, and a thick wool blanket. She didn't say a word to us, and we didn't push any questions on her. We requested of Central if we could get a backup with a female EMT, preferably one who spoke Spanish. It turns out 12–Bravo was in service, and the crew was Mary and Rosa, two excellent EMT's, we knew well.

By the time they arrived, we had the patient on our stretcher, and in the rig. Rosa came on board, and spoke in Spanish to our patient. The girl slowly answered. We figured she had some heroin on board, but we didn't start an IV, or give her narcan. We made the patient as comfortable as possible, and Rosa stayed in the back of the rig with me, as we took a slow easy ride down to Metropolitan hospital, and met up with PD.

Jason and I made our way back uptown, through Spanish Harlem. I was appreciating a lot of the graffiti, in that area, and thought there's a lot of talented artist down here. It's a shame these guys never get recognition, and even get in trouble for trying to express themselves. We made the turn onto 125th street, and I noticed the style of art had changed as we got further uptown, but the storefronts were just as beautiful, and carefully painted, only by a different culture. I became very familiar with the similarities and differences between Latin and African American street art. Then I realized I had distracted myself in a positive way, from the visions and issues of my immediate present.

My thought process was quickly interrupted, as the radio sends us over to One–Two–Eight and Douglas for an abdominal pain. I start bitching about doing a BLS job, and sure enough, we get a thirty-one year old woman who's constipated. She hasn't gone to the bathroom in a couple of days, and now her stomach hurts bad, and she wants to go to the hospital. So I whispered to Jason, "let me borrow 75 cents, I'll buy her a bar of chocolate Ex-Lax and RMA her." Anyway, when I'm done with the paperwork, Jason says to me, "sometimes you need a good taxi job, just to get some brain cells back."

When we get back in service, we're sent up to One–Two–Five and Broadway, for a pediatric asthmatic, a frail nine-year old boy that we both know from the address and apartment number. This will be a real job.

The apartment is on the twelfth floor; we had both been there before. In the lobby, the usual crowd was hitting the pipe. The elevator was taking forever, and one of the teenagers in the crowd was acting stupid. I don't know exactly what he was saying, but I heard someone tell him, "yo blood, stop geekin'—it's coming." So I figured they just want to hit the pipe, and when the elevator comes, I'm thankful to enter their makeshift urinal.

When we get upstairs, I find our patient, who's really tight. He woke up and couldn't breathe. He wasn't able to complete sentences, and was working very hard to move any air. So Jason sets up a nebulizer and pulls the reservoir off a non-rebreather mask. He attached the nebulizer to the mask, and I kicked the oxygen bottle up to eight liters a minute. I drew up .2 milligrams of epinephrine, and gave the kid a sub Q injection. His breathing immediately started improving, as we packaged him in the stair chair and headed down to the rig. When we got downstairs, the guys in the lobby must have been feeling real good. One of them starts talking loud to us saying, "EMS, you guys are all right, keep up the good work." Then he continues to his buddy saying, "they ain't cops, they're all right." And we were smiling as we wheeled the kid out of the building, then headed down Broadway, to St. Luke's.

We took the rig over to the bagel store over on One–Ten, when we were done with the kid. We actually got a bit of a break, and didn't get another job until sunrise. We get called over to One–Five–Five and the Hudson River for a drowning. An early morning jogger called in that someone was floating in the river. We get there and we have to drive a little ways through the park, but eventually, we're led down to the rocks, and we find a male body, about twenty, bobbing between the raised stones, out on the water.

We let Central know that we're on the scene, and a few seconds later Brendan came up on the air, and asked if we had a drowning over there. I responded "no, I think he's just been doing the back stoke for the past twelve days." This made Jason laugh, and Brendan cruised by our scene to get a look at him.

We knew who this was. The kid was in the newspaper all week, as there had been a major search going on for him. Anyway, I get out on the rocks, and as the sun is rising above the GW Bridge, I notice that the sea creatures are no different than animals, and they had eaten his eyes. This guy was real bloated, and there were two holes in his face, where his eyes had been.

We had to remove him from the water on a stokes basket, because if you would have tugged on the body to get it out of the water, it would have just come apart, like a chicken in the soup.

So I'm taking part in the social gathering, and enjoying the gallows humor. Brendan tells me he was laughing so hard at my backstroke crack, he almost crashed his vehicle. So the sun is up, and ESU is getting the body out of the water, when we hear 12–Bravo get a call for a major MVA, on Nine–Six, and the Hudson River Drive. As the cops are screaming for an ETA, me and Jason are a forty-five second straight run away, up the highway.

Jason gets on the air, and says to Central, "6–Victor, I have an 83 here, left with PD, put me on the pin job." We're assigned to the MVA, and fly down the highway, towards the accident. We get there even before Mary and Rosa arrived. When I saw the car, I couldn't believe this guy was still alive. Not only that, he was still alert. The car had been cut off by a speeding taxicab. It went off the highway, and into the drainage ditch. It rolled a few times and stopped upright against the wall that divides the highway from the Riverside Drive promenade. Anyway, I can't believe this guy wasn't decapitated. His head went through the windshield, and his body was over the steering wheel and still in the car. He had a tremendous gash over his eye that oozed blood like a sink faucet. I put pressure on it with my thumb, then had to pinch the wound shut, because my whole thumb went inside it.

I was thinking this guy was only a couple of minutes away from bleeding out. The firemen quickly cut away the broken windshield, and with Jason's help, had him on a long board, in less than three minutes.

St. Luke's was literally, only two minutes away. I drove, and Jason was in the back. I don't know how he did it, but when I backed into the emergency room ambulance bay, the guy had two sixteens in him, running wide open, and Jason was pumping an IV bag up with the BP cuff.

We came out to finish our paperwork, while I calmly explained to our backup, that if we dilly-dallied on the scene trying to put a KED on this patient, like they wanted to, we would have brought in a well-immobilized hypovolemic corpse.

I treated Jason to a coffee on the way back for the tour change. I told him he hit those lines like a champion, and showed him the paperwork. The whole job, from the time we were assigned, till we were in the hospital, took only nine minutes. We thought this was awesome, as I continued, any other place, any other time, this guy would have been dead.

When we got back to the station, I was calling Jason Simba, the Line King. I drove home, and was thinking that with the right partner, fucked-up awesome nights, would become a regular thing.

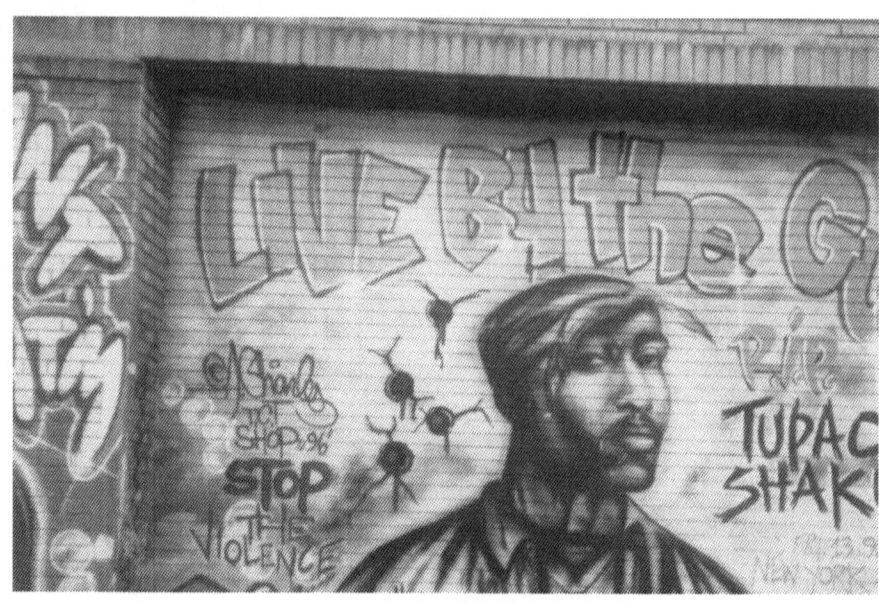

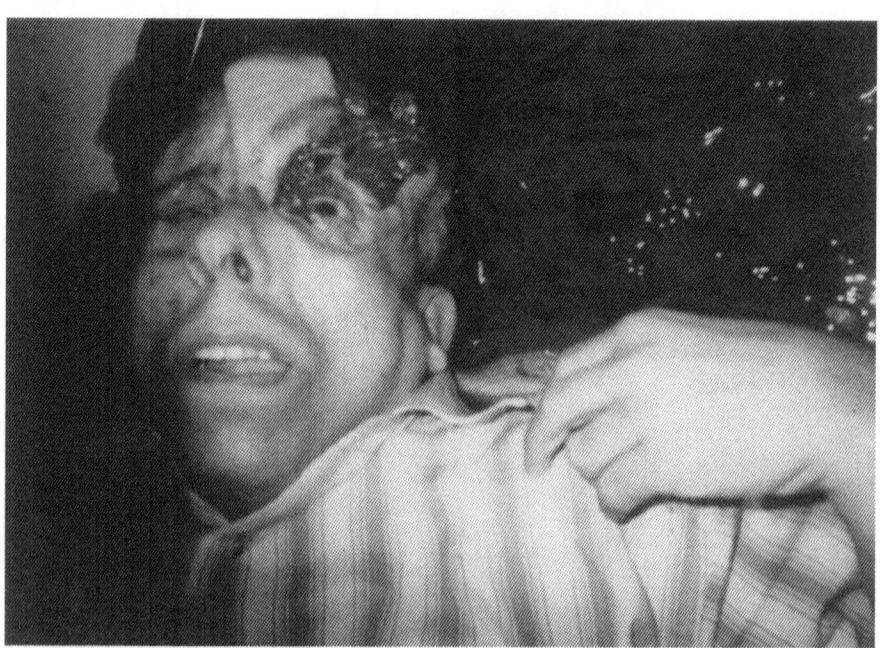

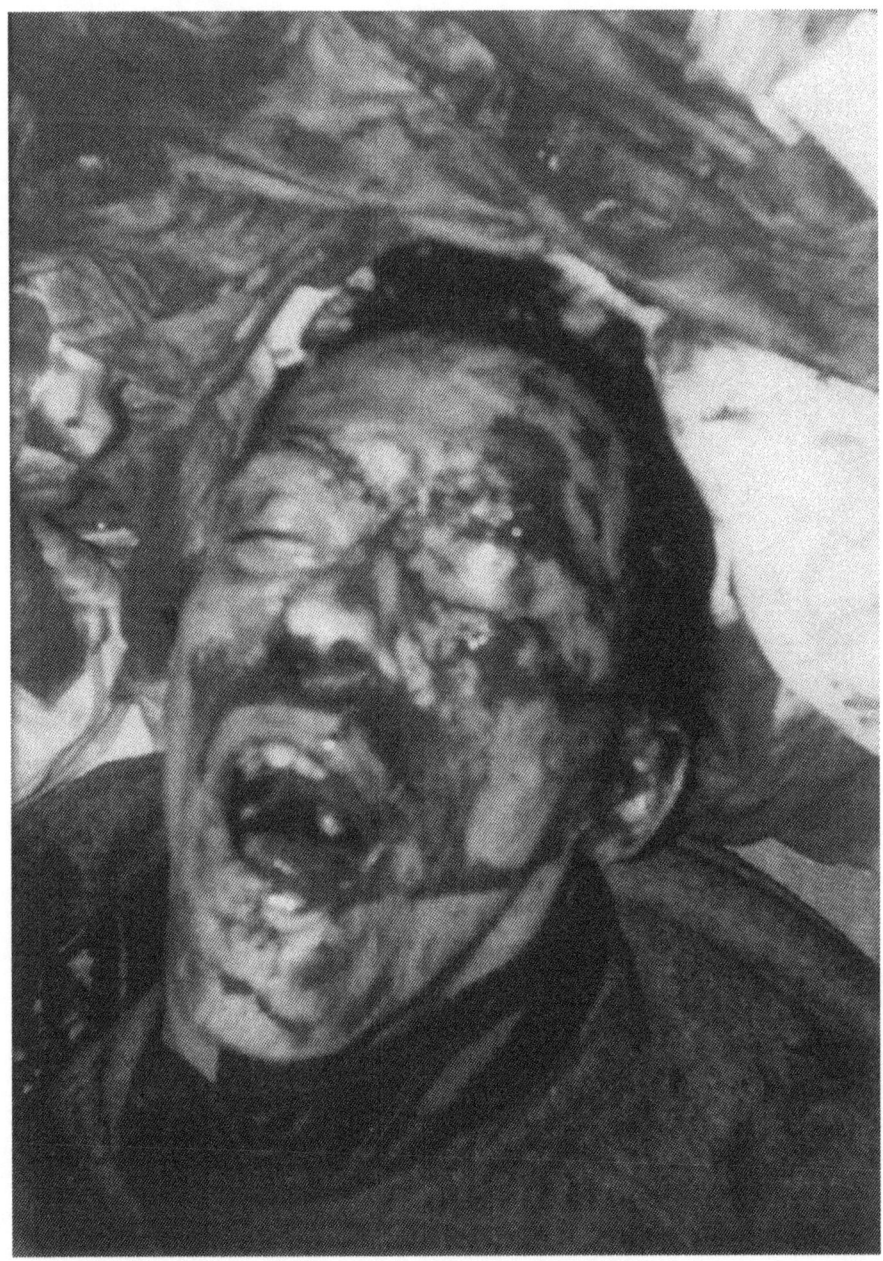

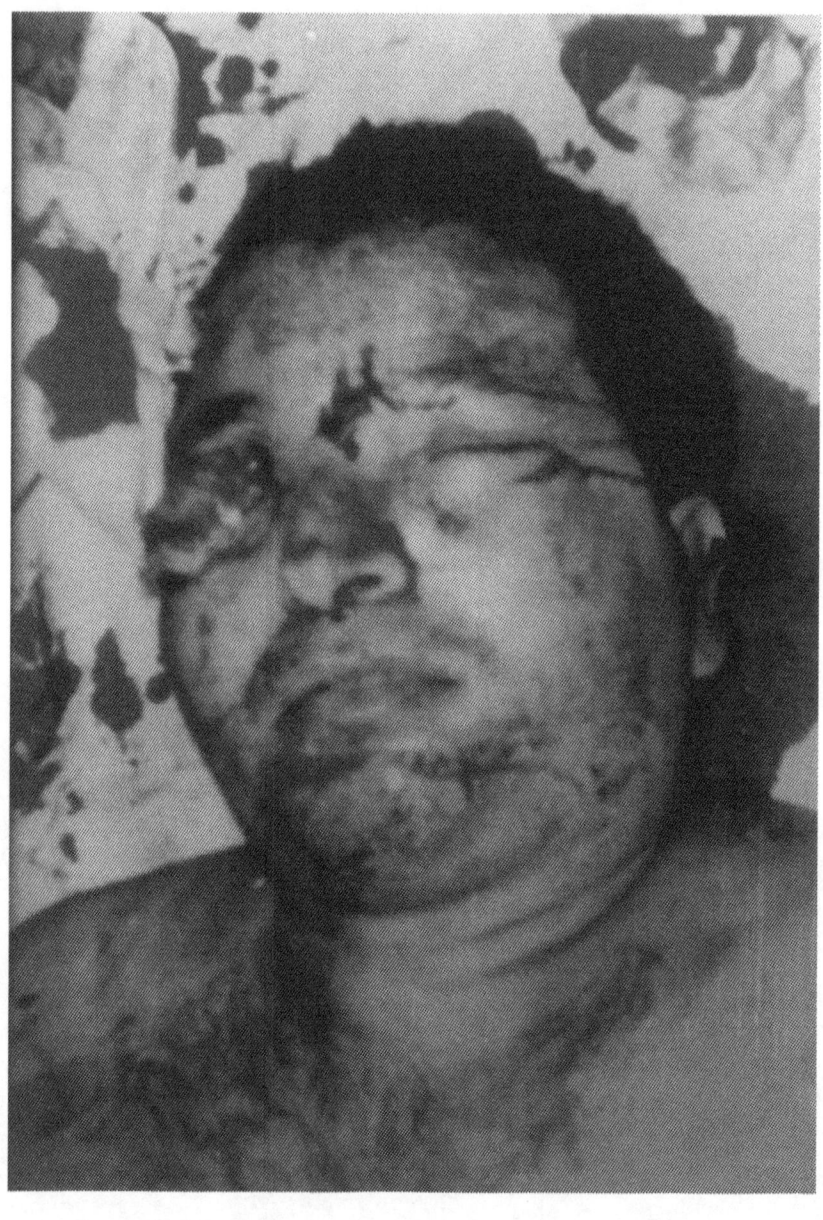

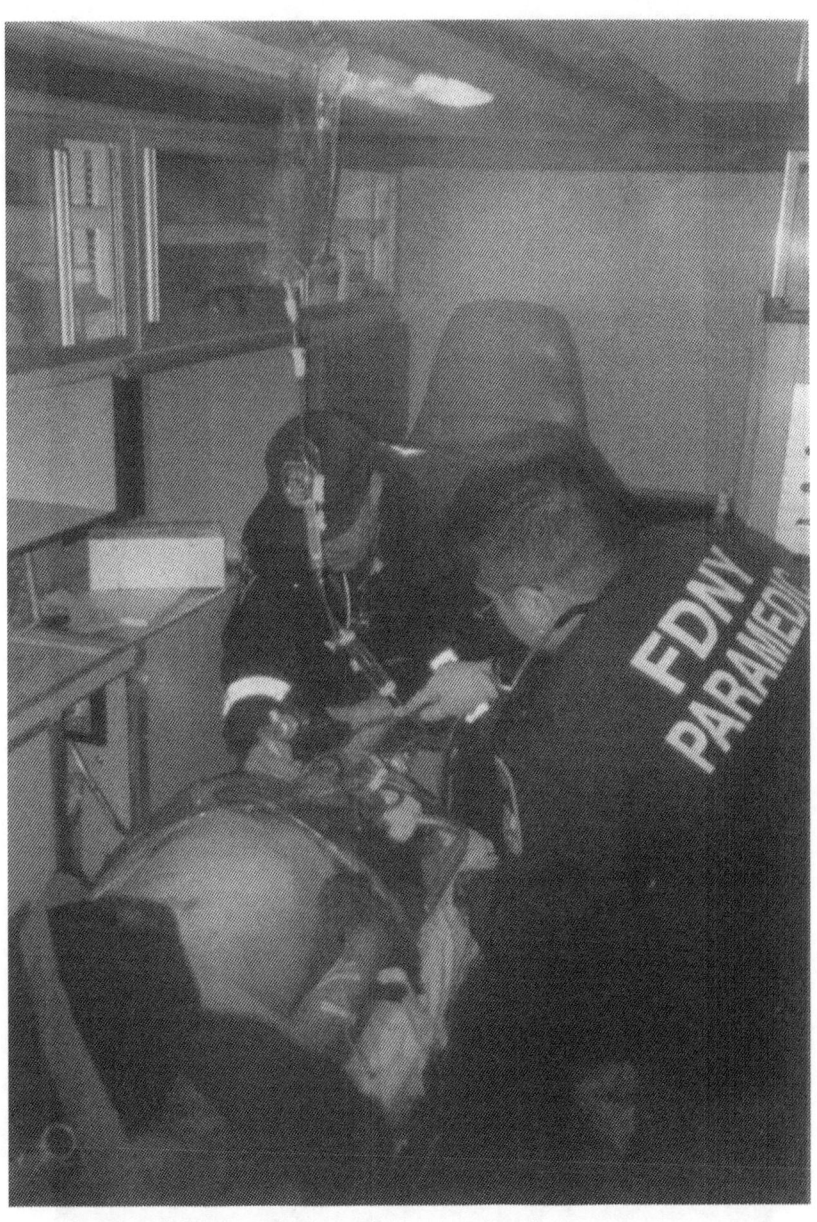

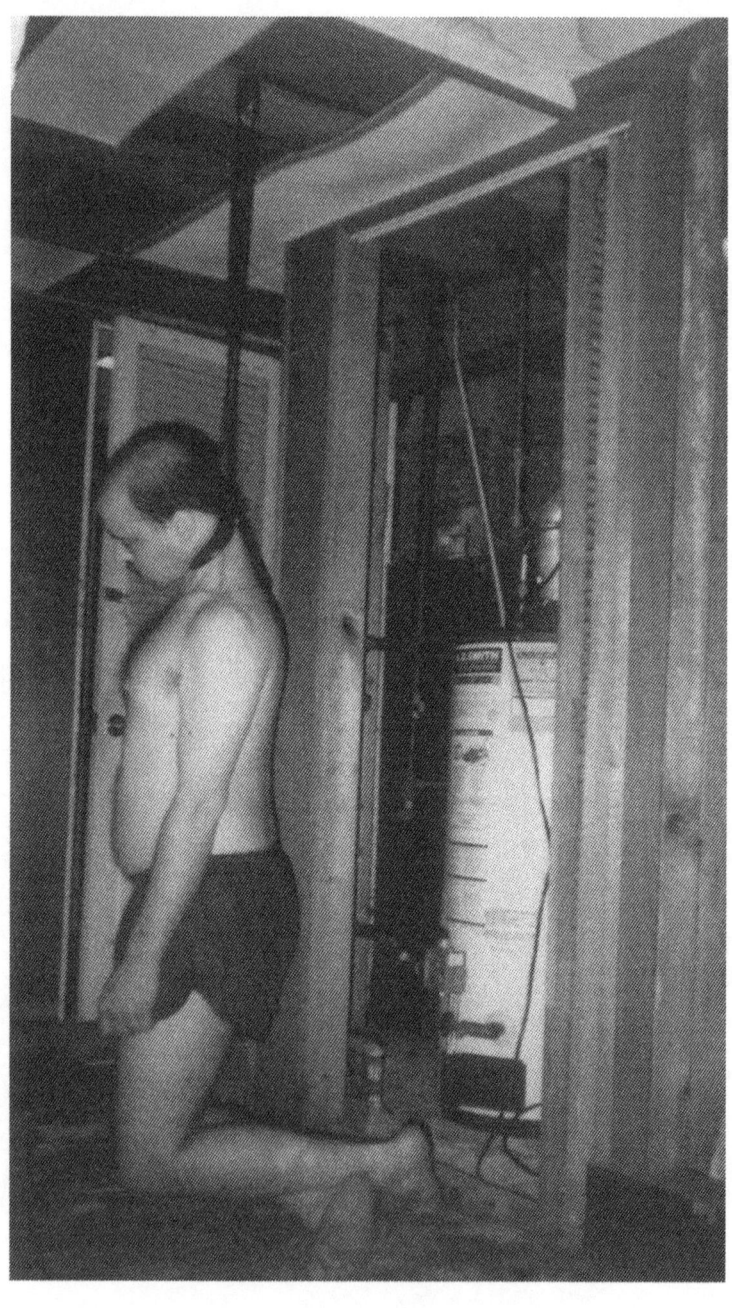

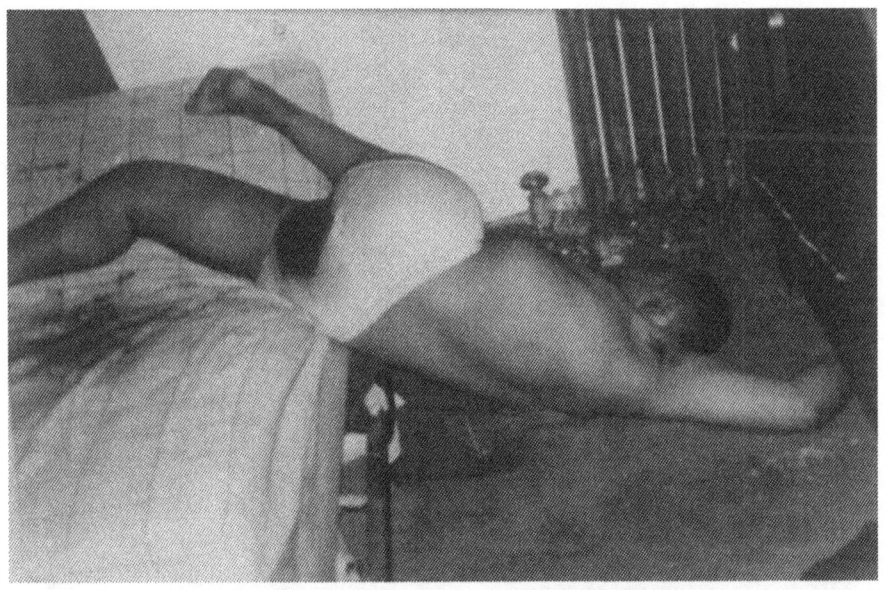

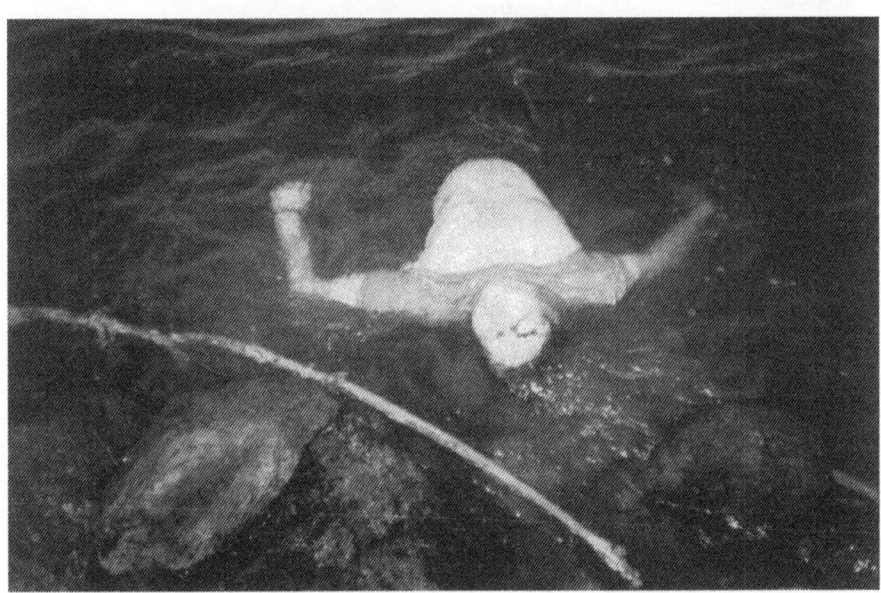

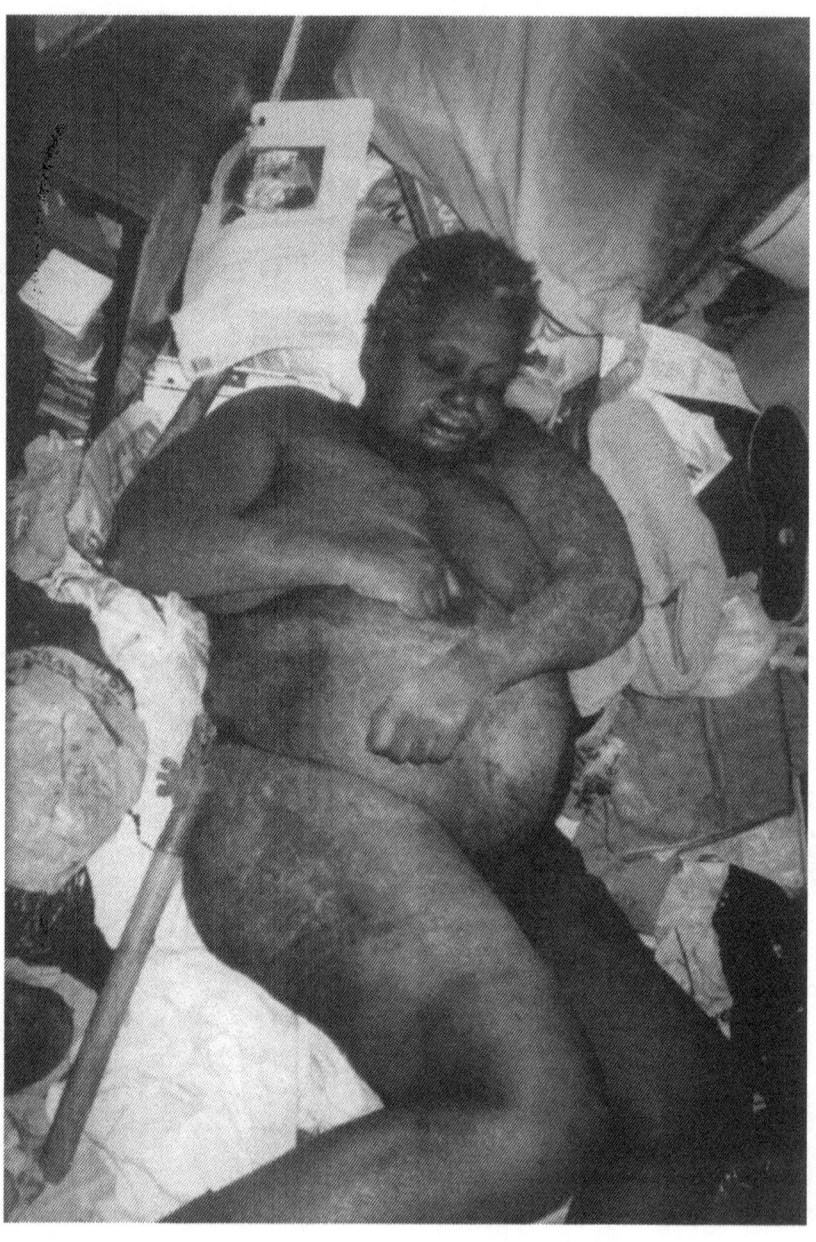

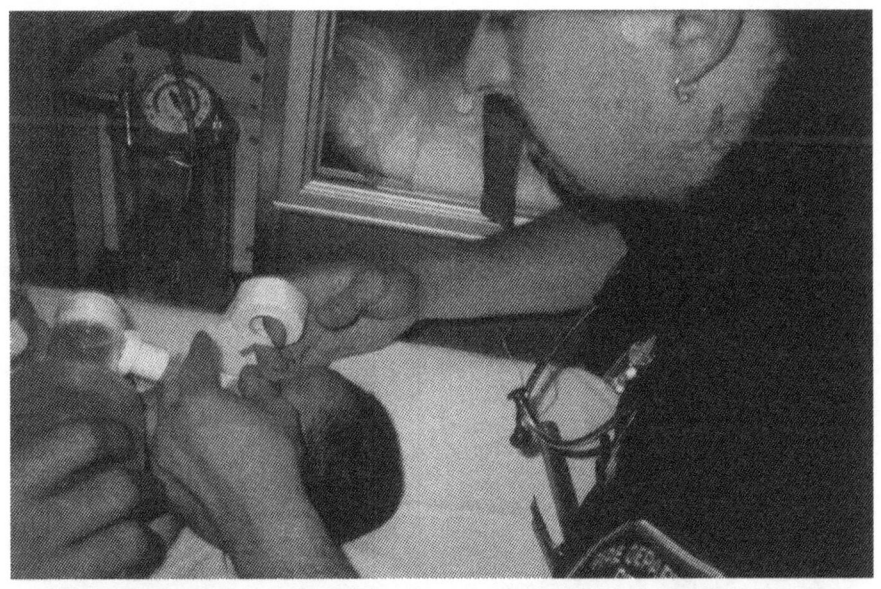

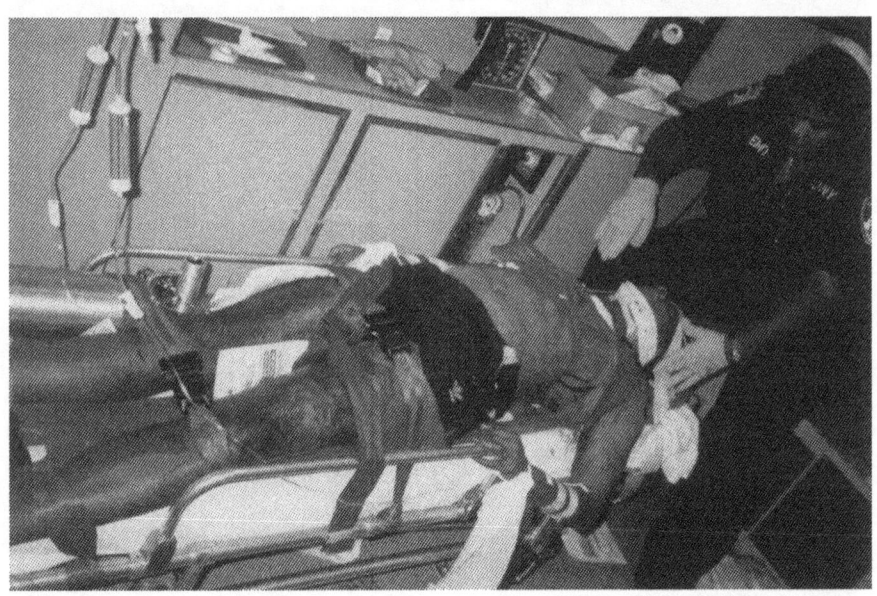

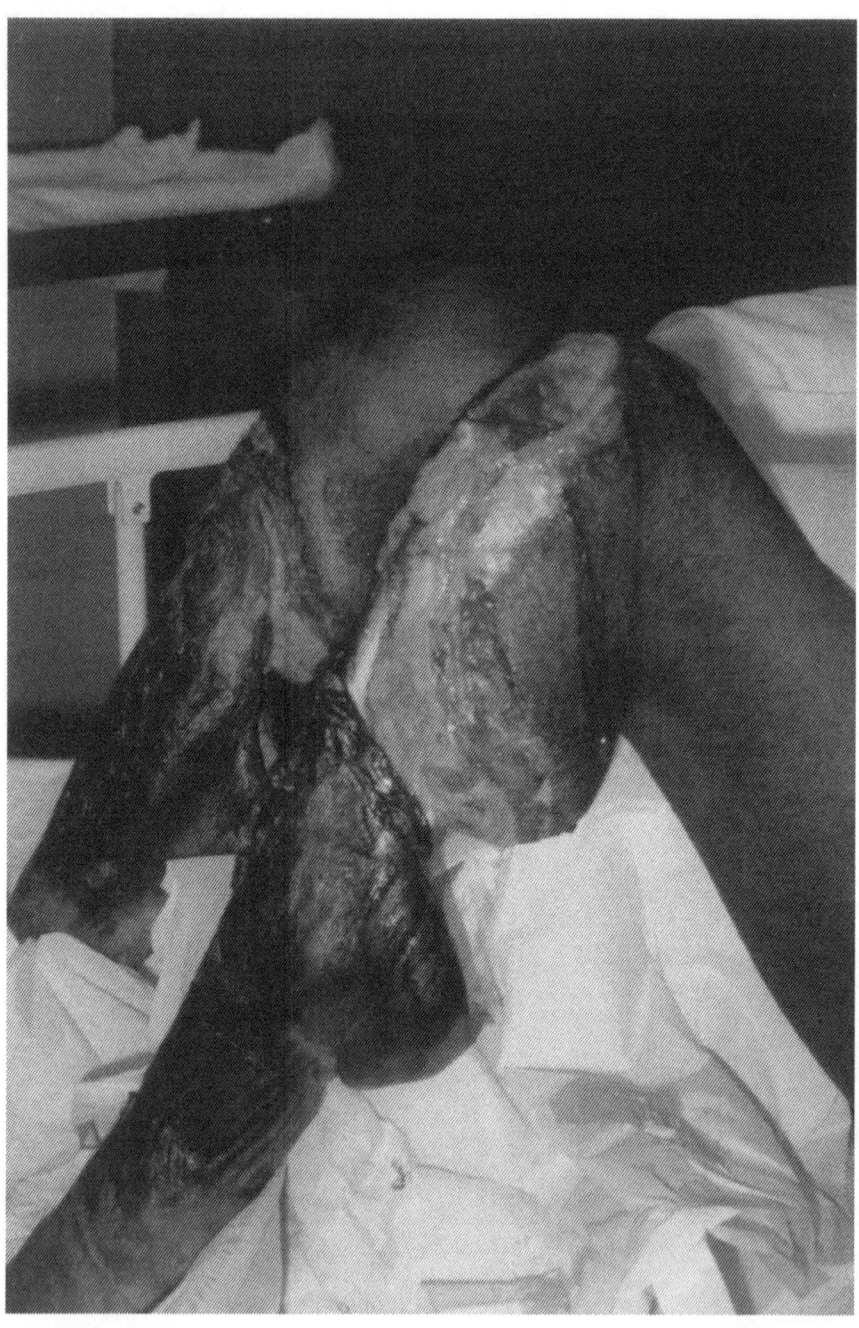

CHAPTER 17

Working on 16–Victor steady is feeling real good. I got excellent partners, and I'm starting to establish an identity. I really believe it's our unit and I take personal pride in keeping it running, and pulling our weight. No one has to pick up my jobs, and we never hold a signal. We go from 63 to 98 (assigned to back in service), in under 20 minutes consistently on bullshit street-jobs.

I hate getting mandated, and I know the only way around this is to pick up a lot of overtime on tour 3. I recently got in trouble because I refused a mandate. I'm saying to my lieutenant, "let me get this right, I come to work, and because I've got child care responsibilities during the day, and I'm not going to work somebody else's hours, I'm going to lose three days pay for being insubordinate, while so-and-so bangs out and gets a full day's sick pay, for staying home." So I understand the policy, come to work get fucked, what else should I expect? Anyway, this pissed me off good, and mandates around the station, both BLS and ALS, were keeping morale low. I was determined to do overtime on my own terms; besides, I liked a lot of the guys on tour three. So I was volunteering on the evening units regularly, and on a lot of those days there were double vacancies open, so Jason would come in early too.

Brendan, being the smart guy that he was, caught wise to what we were doing, and he also started grabbing a lot of evening overtime. This was pissing off the morning lieutenants, because a lot of times they didn't have enough people to mandate.

So it's a nice day to work, not too hot, not too cold. I'm turning the double play on Victor with Jason tonight, starting at four, then rolling the unit over at midnight. We get out of the box quick, and we're hit with a job over on Edgecombe and One–Four–Five, for a burn. A twenty-one year old girl had been hanging out. She said she was jumped by three other girls, who kicked her ass, and poured a gallon of bleach over her head. She had gotten back to her building, and someone helped her up to her apartment, where she called 911. The girl couldn't see anything. She was only able to distinguish light from dark. We instructed her mother to run the shower, and we cut all her clothes off. She had a lot of blisters and rashes all over her upper body, neck and arms. Her mother helped us get her showered off, then we wrapped her up, and gave two drops of proparacaine in each eye. I continued to flush her eyes with sterile water, en route to Harlem Hospital. When we were done, I asked Jason if he thought we were going to have a full moon tonight. "It's sure starting out like that, isn't it," he responded, as he pushed the 98 button that would let Central know we were ready for the next assignment.

We were hanging out by the ambulance bay, and bullshitting with Sy. He'd just been discharged from the hospital again, after another bout with pneumonia, and was waiting to get cleared by the medical department to go back to work. We find out a lot of the guys are going to barbecue tonight, and he tells us when we get a break, we should stop back at the station. So Central calls us and sends us up to Convent Avenue for a difficulty breathing, as Sy says to us, he's going to go get some meat, and start cleaning the gas grill.

So we get up on the forth floor of the building, there's no elevator, and of course, our forty-eight year old female is well over 200 pounds. She's giving us the I-yi-yi's, and I'm thinking she does look a little pale. She was also cool and moist, and saying she was dizzy. Her pressure was 180/100, and she told us the only medication she takes is verapimil. So she goes on the monitor, and her heart rate is like her weight, well over two hundred.

I hit a good line in her right antecubital vein, and Jason and I set her up for an adenosine bolus. I drew up 6 milligrams in a syringe, and Jason drew 10 cc's of saline out of the IV bag. We agreed that we would push our chemical cardioversion on three. I took the low port on the line, and Jason took the high port, with the flush. He clamped off the tubing above our syringes, and I counted, "one two three." I shot the adenosine into her vein, as Jason quickly flushed the line with his push.

I watched the patient and the monitor…nothing. About thirty seconds passed, and we knew we had to try again. This time I loaded 12 milligrams into the syringe, and we prepared to go again. I counted three, and we pushed the drug, and the saline into our patient…still no conversion. The lady was still telling us she was dizzy, and now her chest hurt. We would only get one more chance at this, and then I would have to call for orders that would have involved sedation, and electro-cardioversion.

I really didn't want to do this if I didn't have to. I drew up another 12 milligrams of adenosine into my syringe. Jason took another 10 milligrams of saline from the bag, and we got ready for our last try. Before the push, I was expecting it wouldn't work again, and I asked, "if it doesn't work, do you want me to ask the doctor for morphine or Valium, when I call for the cardioversion order?" He just said to me, like he'd done this job already, "don't worry, it's going to work this time." We inserted our needles into the tubing and I counted one – two – three. We pushed the drug, and I again watched the patient and the monitor. All of a sudden, she clenched her chest as her eyes bulged out real big, and her mouth opened wide, like a silent scream, as nothing came out.

The monitor was recording for us, and when I looked down it was in the process of recording about 6 seconds of flat-line. We knew this was going to happen, but it still freaked me out when it did. Just as sudden as it stopped, her heart started again, and stabilized at 88. Her blood pressure went down to 130/82, and if I didn't know we did a good job, I did when she gave me a bear hug, and was saying, "oy poppy, you saved my life, thank-you, thank-you." We knew it wasn't a big deal, but this woman loved us. She really believed we saved her life, and it felt good.

Down on the rig, Jason told me, "if she calls you poppy chulo one more time, I'm going to puke." I said, "I don't even know what a poppy chulo is," and he responded, "good, cause you'd be unbearable if you did." Whatever it meant, it made my back feel a little better, after carrying her down the four flights.

It was a short ride up to CPMC, and when the assignment is complete, we go across the street to the stick-em-up deli, and get a couple of coffees. We hear a job for a shooting go over the PD radio, in the Colonial Park houses, off the FDR Drive. It's up on the twentieth floor, and I suggest to Jason, "why don't we cruise down that way, and see what's up?" I don't even get to finish the sentence, as we were already moving in that direction, just a bit faster than cruising speed. Low and behold, we get called for the shot, and since we had a quick start, we were already on the drive, heading south, as we let Central know we would be at the scene in thirty seconds.

When we get into the lobby, you could tell something happened by the hectic activity. People are asking, "what happened," and "where are we going?" Other guys are saying, "someone got shot up on twenty." Which was correct, but we don't confirm that. So everyone piles into the elevator with us, and the cops. We push twenty, and others think nothing of hitting floors below us. So we stop at 10—11—14—16, etc. We finally get to twenty, and step out into the hall, to find two guys, each shot in the ass. One guy is twenty-four. He's lying on his belly yelling in pain, and his pants are covered with blood. The other guy is thirty, and he's about 8 feet further down the hall. He's laying in a fetal position, and is expressing no comfort since he's been shot once in the ass, and out his side.

I take the first guy, and Jason has the second. By now our backup is down in the lobby, and we ask them to bring up two boards. So I cut the guys pants off, and unfortunately, I have to cut his Daffy Duck boxers off too. He's got one entrance wound, in his left ass cheek, and it exits out the front femur. He's got a second entrance wound in the right ass cheek, with no exit wound, and this is where a lot of blood loss is coming from.

Jason is telling me his guy ain't too bad, and his blood pressure is still over 110. My guy is losing a lot of blood, and I use veniguards to occlussively seal his gunshot wounds. I dropped two sixteen's in him, and got him ready for transport. By this time Jason had his guy ready, and the vertical urinal was waiting. So we're going down, and of course the elevator stops. We ask the guy, "take the next one please," and he looks around quickly and says "no problem," as he steps back. It stops again at 13, and again I ask the person waiting, "please take the next one."

Now consider, we got two guys shot, on boards, and IV'd, with all of our equipment. We have two cops, two EMT's and two medics, all crammed into this small, smelly, piss-filled elevator. Well this genius tells me, "fuck you," and tries to push his way into the elevator, while making forceful physical contact with one of the officers. This cop took his nightstick, and jammed it right under this guy's sternum, then pushed him out into the hall, and up against the wall. The other cop stepped out, and the elevator door closed behind him, and we proceeded down. I looked across at Jason, and said "it's a shame this guy is so fucked-up, I would have liked to stay and watch that."

So when we get down to the lobby, there's like ten more cops there. They step into the elevator as soon as we're out, and head up to thirteen. We put one patient in each rig, and split up with BLS, taking a quick run down to Harlem. Afterwards, we're back in service, restocked, and ready to continue serving the community.

We did a few really annoying, bullshit, abuse of the system, taxi jobs, and it was well into the evening when we brought another upper respiratory infection to Harlem Hospital. When we were out in the ambulance bay, I saw Sy, and he gave me a couple of hamburgers for us. Then he started to tell me that the cops brought someone over to the ER, to be identified by our shooting victims. It turns out, these guys were shot by a woman who lived in the building, as he continued, "see, you really got to watch who you fuck with around here." We went on with our tour, and rolled back up to our area where we sat about 10 minutes, before we got sent on another assignment. This would be our last job before we went back to the station to pick up a student, who would ride with us on the overnight.

We get sent up to One–Six–O and Fort Washington Avenue, for an unconscious on the street. When we get out of the rig, I see this guy who is out cold on the sidewalk, and some idiot is on top of him trying to do CPR. This would be OK, except Hector was doing CPR on a guy who had a strong pulse, and was breathing well. So Jason says to me, "this guy's got pinpoint pupils and a big lump on his forehead," which I had already noticed.

I went back to the rig, and grabbed a board and collar. I'm asking people in the crowd that's hanging over us, to "please step back," and "I think he's going to be all right." Well our hero is telling people, "see, I saved his life, see," and he's pushing the crowd back away from us, which was good. Anyway, we're in the back of the bus, and I ask Jason, "how many ribs to you think got broke by that douche bag," as I felt for flail segments, or deformity. Jason hit a line, and we gave 2 milligrams of narcan, one amp of dextrose, and 100 milligrams of thiamin. So nothing is happening, and we decide our coma-cocktail needs a little extra kick. So we give him another two mgs of narcan, and our boy wakes up.

He starts going wild, as he tears out the IV, and is climbing off the board and stretcher. We had to tie him down with cravats, and the whole ride up to CPMC, he's trying to spit on me, and is cursing me out, as I'm thinking, I should have let Hector do CPR on you another 10 minutes or so.

So we finish our paperwork, and head back to the station. It's after midnight now, and we meet our student. He's a Navy Seal from Texas, named Chad. He was a big guy, and was impatient while waiting for us. We introduced ourselves, and apologized for being on a late job. I told him it was busy, and that he would get plenty of work tonight. He responded to me that he knew this, and other guys that rode with us said they felt like barbarians who ate raw octopus with their bare hands, after a night on 16–Victor. He added that we were the only unit he wanted to ride with. This was very flattering, and I reassured him, that nothing would go down tonight, that we wouldn't get a piece of.

We get in service and try to head down to the bagel store. We didn't get there; we got hit with a job for a difficulty breathing. The text stated—75-year-old female, history of diabetes, cardiac, CVA, and hypertension. I say to Chad, these jobs are the norm, and we'll see what else the night brings. So we get on the scene, and go into a small, well-kept apartment. We find a woman over 300 pounds, in bed. She's pretty comatose, and the family tells us she's non-verbal, but usually more awake. Anyway, she's incontinent, fecal and urine, and hasn't been changed in a while. A good long while. The smell is enough to make your eyes start tearing, and it surely cleared all the sinuses in the room. So the patient is basically paralyzed from a previous stroke. She's a double amputee, below the knees, and a tube-feeder. She's hot and soaked in sweat. I heard her gurgling very rough sounding wet breathing, and asked Chad what he believed to be wrong with the patient. He replied he thought we had pulmonary edema, but we didn't agree, as Jason explained she's probably an aspiration pneumonia.

She didn't have any good veins, but we told Chad to see if he could hit a line on her. He and Jason each took a shot at it without success. We cleaned up the patient as well as possible, and trying to get her on the stretcher was like moving lethargic Jell-O. I saw Chad was turning a nice shade of green, and was ready to chuck. In the elevator, Jason is asking if he's OK, and he nods yes. I looked over at him, and asked, "son, when was the last time you sniffed a 40 pound diaper?" He was really working hard, at not vomiting, and he spoke slowly, "Dan, I can handle any trauma you got, but I've never been around this before." So I broke the good news, that he would be in the back with me, and we still needed to get a line. Her poor venous access hadn't miraculously changed in the last five minutes, and I tried one stick along her thumb with a 22. Chad tried once more on her other hand, but we couldn't get a line. While we were in the ER, I introduced Barbara, the charge nurse, to our student. She asked us to help her move the patient onto the bed, and get her undressed.

When we got the diaper off this woman, she had a giant bedsore on her butt, that you could put a fist into. It was stuffed with gauze and hadn't been changed in days. Barbara started to pull the infected cling out of this oozing wound, and that was all she wrote. Chad flew over to the sink, as the smell of rotten flesh tore the puke out of him. He was gagging over the sink, splashing his face with cold water, as Jason went over and gave him a pat on the back, and said we were back in service.

We go across the street to the station, and the boys got the barbecue going to full effect. Sy is holding court over there, and he gives us some grilled chicken that was out of this world. By now I was really starving, as Chad said to me, "I don't know how you guys do that every day." He wasn't quite ready to eat yet, but it didn't matter because we were already getting another job.

We get sent all the way up to Academy Avenue, for an OB comp. I'm saying this is probably a taxi job, as we're heading up the drive. When we get to the building, we're met by a frantic Spanish guy, about 23 or so. He's telling us, "my wife, my wife." Jason asks as we're walking in, "what's that matter with your wife, sir?" "She's having a baby, hurry, hurry," he says. So when we get up the stairs, the cops tell us she's going to deliver. We go into the bedroom, and a woman about 21, is naked on the bed, and screaming in labor. I say to Chad, "do you really want us showing up in the middle of the night to deliver your baby?"

Jason takes a look, and sees that the baby is crowning. The woman's water broke that morning, and she was having contractions all day. "So I guess now was a good time to call an ambulance," I say to Jason, as her contractions are like 20 seconds apart. So Jason decides he's going to deliver, and I'm following his lead. I'm off to the side, and with that last big push, the inevitable exploding diarrhea impacted on him all over his waste and legs. We let Chad cut the cord, and suction the baby, and after cleaning up the mother and newborn, started down to the rig. I let him start a line on the mother, and he was really impressed when the placenta delivered.

Jason got himself cleaned up a bit at CPMC, and we then went out of service, decon. Back at the station, Jason got changed, and finished cleaning up, while I went back to the grill for more food. We were talking about babies being delivered and Sy's telling us about one he did a while back, where the woman was on the bowl when they walked in, and she delivered the baby into the toilet. I liked talking with Sy, and the other old timers, and I gave them a lot of respect. When Jason came back, the boys were getting on him good, and they were telling him it didn't matter if he showered, the cats were still going to follow him around all night.

We were back in service, and Chad was feeling a lot better. We told him we would listen to the PD radio, and try to find some trauma for him. While cruising around the area, Chad decides he wants to get a soda. So we pull over by an all-night bodega. I realize he's getting a little bit of culture shock, when I see him getting frustrated by the locked store door. I point out the little cutout slot at the end of the bulletproof window where the guy would take your money, and then bring you a soda, or whatever else you might need.

13–Charlie gets an assignment for a male assaulted. It's not too far, so we'll just cruise by. Besides, it's a street job. We head up One–Four–Five, and up over the hill to Amsterdam. By this time Ziffy and Derrick are there. They have a crack-head who got his ass kicked, inside the donut store. He had a nice fat bloody lip, and was scratched up good around his neck and arms. But this wasn't anything we were really looking for. So I told them to be safe, and we would meet up with them later.

The night is moving on. We get a job over in Mt. Morris Park, for an unconscious. Jason looks back, and says to Chad, "these jobs could be anything from a guy sleeping, to a DOA." We find our patient on a bench, out for the count, with the tight pinpoint pupils. And of course, he's pissed himself. So we scrape him off the bench, and onto our rig. We let the student hit a line, and explained why we would give the drugs that would help our patient. "Not too much narcan," I said, "because it makes a lot of problems involving vomit and withdrawal." So Chad gives the magic wake-up juice, we call vitamin-N. This guy becomes alert, and he's still drunk, but happy. He's asking us, "who are you," and laughing, as he starts singing. So we ask him, "don't you know any good songs?" He's still laughing, and he starts singing Old McDonald had a farm. So I'm having a good time with this job, and I'm saying to him, "no, no, you got the words wrong." I get him to start singing, "old McDonald did some her-ron, E-I-E-I-O."

Chad is cracking up, and I hear Jason up front laughing too. We get to the emergency room, and as we come out of the back of the rig, our patient is saying "hi" to everyone we see. And all the way to the nurse, he's singing "old McDonald did some her-ron, E-I-E-I-O." So we get to triage, and Barbara says to me " you guys always leave 'em singing and laughing, don't you," as she bends over our patient and asks, "how much her-ron did old McDonald do?" She then scribbled on my ACR, and while kicking us out of the emergency room, asked "do me a favor, take the next one over to St. Luke's, please." I said we'll see what we can do, and when we went out by the station, we could see the barbecue crew still kicking back.

Sy was becoming concerned because they still had a lot of food left, but they were running out of charcoal, and all the propane was long gone. The sun would be up soon, and we still wanted to get Chad some good work, if possible. We had the PD radio on, scanning uptown in the Three–Four precinct. I told Jason I felt like we had been working a week already, and he looked at his watch, and replied "no, only fourteen hours."

We heard 13–X-ray get a job for a fire standby; a car burning on the Henry Hudson Parkway, up by Dykeman Street. We knew Tom hated these jobs, and we figured it would be good to hang out, and watch the firemen extinguish it. I asked Jason if he wanted to pick up the job for them, and he said, "yeah, what the fuck." So he tells Central we're right by the highway, and we could be there faster if X-ray wants us to pick up that job. Tom said, in a tired voice over the radio, "take it," and he thanked us. So we went up the FDR Drive, under the large white buildings that lead to the bridge, and around and up the parkway. We could see a lot of firemen near the car, as we approached, more than was normal. They had just gotten there, and the car was still burning. It was parked off the shoulder of the highway, and the flames were shooting up about thirty feet high.

As it turns out, there were two men in the back of a flaming Pathfinder. They had both been handcuffed behind the back, shot in the head, and left in the back of the vehicle, which was then soaked with gasoline and torched. When the fire was out, these guys were crusty. I mean all that was left were charred skeletons. I told Chad that this was probably over drugs, and definitely done to send a message. He was stunned looking at the roasted corpses. I glanced over at Jason, and I mumbled, "he looks like the crypt keeper, from that horror show." And Jason said back, "fuck that, they look like two hamburgers Sy forgot on the grill."

Anyway, this was an awesome crime scene, and we even made all three major news programs, for this one. To this day, these bodies were so fucked up they were never identified. When we went back to the station, Chad still hadn't done any major work, but he was amazed at the night he had, and wanted to do more rotations with us.

So I'm going home, and I see Sy and a lot of the boys are still grilling. I make a comment about just seeing some of his hamburgers on the parkway, and he tells me, "come here and make fun of my cooking, motherfucker." So I go over and hang for a few minutes. I'm so tired I know I'm going to pass out when I go home, so I might as well eat something now. The problem is, these lunatics ran out of charcoal, and now they were using flares, off the vehicles, to cook with. So I say to Sy, "I don't think this is one of your brighter ideas." "I think I'll have to pass on the flare burgers."

When I got back that night, I found out almost everyone on tour 2 got mandated, because anyone who ate a morning hamburger got sick big time, and had to bang out, as the legend of Sy's flare-burgers was born.

CHAPTER 18

The summer is coming and I've been looking forward to it. I'm living on Staten Island, but we've been looking at houses and I'll be moving upstate. The commute is over an hour and a half each way but it's different, because I'm not doing the stop and go bullshit for twenty miles. Driving up the Palisades in the early morning of spring, is something very special to me. It allows me to have quiet time alone and no one breaks my balls about smoking. I'm feeling pretty burnt, and I can't see myself doing this past forty cause I think I'll be dead by then. But these mornings, I really appreciate the beautiful roadside scenery, and I can actually forget the insanity and misery for a few minutes every morning, as I smoke my hydro's and listen to Jimi Hendrix or the Grateful Dead.

I cruise down to the City doing sixty all the way, I'm so glad I don't sit in traffic when I commute. Jason's got himself a few days off so I've been working with Brendan and Matt. Sy has got himself medically cleared again, and I'm starting to pick up easy BLS overtime with him when it's available. So working with Brendan has been excellent. We've been getting along well and the two of us together are like two big dogs in the same yard. We both want to lead, he's got seniority but I want his real respect bad and I'm gonna earn it. I can run with him and inside myself I know he believes this.

We were in service on his unit, 13–Willie and we start our night with a difficulty breathing up on Edgecombe Avenue. We get into a third floor apartment and the cops are talking to a very large seventy year old woman. She's sitting in a recliner and you can tell she's working real hard to breathe. The patient is agitated and very combative. So all she's telling us is she can't breathe. We do our vitals and put her on the monitor and this woman is in V-tach. Brendan tries a line and I start to record the wide waves of the disrythmia from our life pack. I go to the other side of the chair and I try to hit a line in her other arm. We both got nothing, she's has no veins and is fighting us all the way. We know we gotta cardiovert her, and we request a backup, being that this woman is really starting to resemble a beached whale and a three flight carry down is inevitable. We both try a second shot at a line. Brendan got a flash, but couldn't get the catheter advanced. So he asks me to call medical control and talk to the Doc, I'm told to cardiovert her without sedation, which isn't gonna be easy. We get her out of the chair and on the floor.

Brendan flags the monitor, and zap—he cardioverts her into V-fib. "Oh shit" he says and I tell the cop, "you know I hate when that happens." I get the BVM and Brendan promptly shocks her from V-fib to asystole. I looked across at him and I whispered "this is just getting better and better isn't it," as I get an 8.0 ET tube ready. So Brendan is doing CPR and I bang the tube, which he quickly confirms. He hands me an epi and an atropine, and I rapidly dumped them both down the tube. I started to secure the tube with tape and Brendan stopped CPR. The patient came back completely. She was now in a clear sinus tach on the monitor, as she started wrestling with me, trying to tear the tube out. We wanted to dump lidocaine down the tube but my chances of tossing lieutenant lard ass, the length of a football field, were better. This patient was really strong. I looked over at the cops who were just standing there, I said, "guys now would be a good time to help us restrain her." But, before they moved, one of them said back to me, "god damn, I hope I'm brawling with two medics, five minutes after I'm dead." It really took all four of us to get her secured, and she succeeded in dislodging the ET tube. So I deflated the cuff, as she pulled it out of her windpipe. Ziffy and Derek backed us up and helped with the carry down. The cops took our equipment, as the four of us needed to haul the patient. This woman cursed us out, the whole way to the hospital, and I was glad I had the monitor strips, because no one believed she was a flat-line, let alone everything else that went down during this job. So we go back to the station, to restock and change the monitor batteries. We leave the station and head uptown as we make the turn up One–Three–Five, to Saint Nick. We get a job with 13–Charlie for an unconscious in the Harlem Sports Bar, up on Broadway.

We know this place is a tittie bar, and I tell Brendan "the EMS, god owed us this one after that last job." Brendan had a big smile as he lit an old cigar stub, and read the text off the KDT that stated, unconscious female twenty- three years old at scene. Ziffy got on the air and told Central he was responding promptly. I came up on the air after him and said 13–Willie was sixty-three responding, then added, "Zif this'll be the first time you'll be on the scene before us." So we get there and we're led into the bar by this giant black bouncer, with a Fu man chu mustache. This place is mongo titties and the bar is packed. The bouncer is pushing a path clear for us and the four of us follow him eagerly to the girls dressing room. It's business, as usual outside the changing area, and there are some really hot women up on the bar stage shakin their money makers. We get into the dressing room, and it's jammed with naked women, and a couple in some slinky little, very inviting underwear. We find a young woman wearing just this tight tiny zebra bikini bottom, out cold on a table. She's soaked with ice water from the bar and she's got pinpoint pupils. So we think we know what we got. A lot of these naked little honey's are very concerned, and are hovering all over and around us. We're really playing it up, and Zif is telling the girls, "she's real bad off," but he thinks maybe we're not too late.

I've seen this job a couple of hundred times by now, and I know we're gonna wake her up with the vitamin N. So the cops are on the scene now, and everyone is fully involved, they're having a ball to, and they're asking the girls to give her air, and move back so we can work. So we're goin' the whole nine yards here. I draw up a shot of glucagon carefully and slowly and Brendan sets up a line, as Zif puts the BVM on her and

Derek pulls the stretcher around. Zif is carrying on a conversation with like four of these babes as he's bagging the patient. He's explaining we got to give a combination of drugs called a coma cocktail to find out what's wrong, and see if its not too late to fix it. After I give the glucagon intramuscularly in the bicep, Brendan hits a line, and I do a chem strip from the blood in the catheter head. We're acting all serious and the girls are getting more nervous watching Brendan draw out the blood tubes. So I load up one-hundred milligrams of thiamin and hand it to Brendan, and he slowly pushes it in. Next we go with the big bristo of dextrose and our audience is silent, watching and waiting for a miracle. Finally I give Brendan a two-milligram bristo jet of narcan and I draw up another milligram in a 3cc syringe. Brendan tells the girls this is the secret ingredient and as he starts to push it, I come around the table and give the one-milligram IM in the other bicep.

Our patient starts stirring. The strippers are getting excited and are squealin' among themselves. A few seconds later, our patient becomes fully awake and alert. We're looking like real heroes and I'm saying to Brendan "this job ain't all bad is it." We start to package the patient for transport and talk to her on the side. She's telling us she doesn't do drugs. She just had a baby a couple of weeks ago, and the strain of working under the hot lights drained her. I said to her, "we think it was probably heroin she did," but if she didn't want to tell us, it was all right. So she says a friend gave her something to sniff for her belly pain and that if her boss found out she OD'd she'd get fired. So as we're taking her out, the bouncer is asking Zif what happened to her. Zif is a good guy, so he went with the program. He told the guy, that she was a diabetic, and the hard work and hot lights dropped her sugar. She was very grateful to us, and we were given passes to the club by the bouncer, as we were loading into the rig for a short run down to Saint Luke's.

We head uptown after going to One–Ten for coffee and bagels. I got my super deluxe onion bagel with cream cheese and lox and Brendan is telling me "that's fuckin gross." "How can you eat that shit?" I told him it was good for my dick and it helped keep me hard for hours. I said, "why do you think all these old men eat them?" "This shit is better then Viagra" and I started laughing cause he was really buying into this.

So we go sit by the graveyard on One–Five–Five and I start to nod out, but Brendan is already snoring like a fuckin' chainsaw. I'm thankful when the radio interrupts us, and sends us up to Fort Tryon, for a choke, backing up 13–Charlie. We're a distance away, and I ask Zif to give us an update when he gets on the scene. Anyway we're still about four minutes out, when Zif gets on the air and tells us to slow it down, he says "it's not a choke but keep it coming cause you gotta see this." So I'm telling Brendan "I think Zif's got a Kodak moment for us," and we keep rolling uptown.

When we get on the scene we got this Dominican woman about forty-five, and she can't speak any English. Her mother called in, because the woman got her denture plate stuck to her tongue. I couldn't figure out how the fuck she pulled this off at three in the morning and she was so nervous she was clearly hyperventilating. I was trying not to laugh, as I told Derek "I think we'll leave her in your capable hands, and take an eighty-seven." Zif told us "Thanks for the back" and I said "No, thank you Mr. Acavono" as we walked out the door and back to our unit.

Its near sunrise, the dead of night, but the radio just keeps goin' and goin' and goin' you know, sorta like that stupid pink bunny. I mention this fact to Brendan and he just mumbles in his best homeboy voice, "you next bro, you next." We listen intently, as our pork chop dispatcher clears her board. Brendan tells me, "the fat bastard probably just woke up and noticed thirty jobs holding," then I added, "And there's lot's of Twinkies to be had." "Every time she screws a unit, one pops out of the console for her."

Anyway, we get sent to the MacCombs Dam Bridge for an MVA. This is right next to Yankee Stadium, and it's one of about five small bridges that separates Harlem from the South Bronx. We start to roll, and I'm telling Brendan, "At least it's a street job, probably just some asshole with allstatitis," and "it'll be a piece of cake." "No chance," he says to me, as he's reading our on board computer screen. "PD is requesting the unit, for one man in custody." So there'll be no way we can RMA him, but we might be able to eighty-four him. We get on the scene, the same time as 13–Charlie, and Zif is thinking like me. He says to me as he steps out of his rig, "I hope this guy isn't bullshit, this way you can transport him." As I approach the vehicle I see this guy pinned in there, and the car is smacked up good on the driver's side, and front end. The windshield is spider webbed from this idiot's head and it looks like a canister of baby powder exploded inside the car. This guy is really acting wild. I ask the cop, "is that what I think it is, all over the car." And he says "there's enough blow in there to turn on Brooklyn."

So TNT, a plainclothes PD unit, started to tail this guy up near 3333 Broadway. He was driving pretty erratically, and they radioed a patrol unit of their location to pull this guy over. By this time he was cruising down One–Five–Five and when he noticed the red lights of a blue and white behind him, he decided to jet.

He headed over toward the Bronx, and all he had to do was get across the bridge, into another Borough, and they would have given up the chase. Apparently this guy had a gallon ziplock back filled with cocaine. The cops told us it was probably a kilo, and it didn't look like there was any reason to doubt this. When he started to try to elude the police, he started to eat it. We think he must've ate like five or six ounces, and when he crashed on the bridge they said he was doing about seventy, as he sideswiped the rail for a couple of hundred feet, before becoming pinned against it. The bag of blow spilled all over the car, as he collided with the bridge. Well, like I said, it was everywhere, all over the patient, the dashboard, and windshield.

When we get him extricated from the vehicle this guy is completely fucked up. It takes seven cops to hold him down and get him tied to the stretcher. It's really true that this stuff alters the mind so, as to give like super human strength for a time. But it's also true that the consequence is death! When we get in the rig, this guy snaps one of the cravats that was holding his arm, and another that was holding a leg down. He's flipping out but at least he's still half restrained. Brendan and I are trying to keep him on the stretcher, and the cop tells us to let him go. He says to the patient "that's it motherfucker your getting lit up." He hits him right on the belly with an electric tazer gun, and this guy is screaming like he's getting off on it. We get him tied again, the patient starts yelling at us, "you're all gonna fuckin' die tonight." "I'm gonna kill all your fuckin' asses." So Brendan starts to cut his clothes off and this guy has got cash everywhere, every pocket on his pants and his shirt is stuffed with twenties, fifties and hundreds. He starts wigging out even more and is still screaming as the cop puts the tazer right on his belly again, the patients back arches up and he's gritting his teeth yelling, "give it to me, give it to me, I like it." I look over at Ziffy and he says, "it's like when King Kong was eating the electrical wires and was getting stronger." Then Brendan said, " yeah, and where's Godzilla when you need him."

We transported this person over to Harlem Hospital as quickly as possible. We were there about ten minutes when this guy went nighty night for good. He wound up being in V-fib for over an hour, before his heart finally quit. After that job I was really keyed up, but I was also physically drained. I was glad the rest of the tour passed quickly, and without another assignment. When we took it back for the change we were still talking about this job, and as I left, I told Brendan "it kinda made you forget about wrestling with Haystacks Calhoun eight hours ago didn't it." He laughed a little and he said, "yeah, but it didn't make me forget about this." As he pulled out a small card that had one of the strippers phone numbers on it. I told him, "You da Man." "I didn't even notice you got it" and he continued "yeah you should see the one Ziffy got" and I said back "wow, now I really feel like shit," as I started to walk towards the parking lot with him.

CHAPTER 19

I'm enjoying my new house, and really liking the ride down to the city. I notice for a lot of the commute my rear view mirror is black, until I start to get close to the city, then I can see a few headlights.

I'm working with Brendan again, and now I really look forward to seeing him. I still piss him off a lot, but at least now I'm not trying to anymore. I don't think he'll admit it to anyone, but I'm starting to feel that he thinks I'm a good partner and a good guy. So this motivates me to really work hard for him, and be a partner he can trust. I make sure I'm on top of my game whenever we're together, and it's good that I do, because we're always busy. And if I fuck up, he won't pull any punches. Nor would I, and this is the way we both want it.

Tonight we're in service on Victor, and we're getting a job before we even have the vehicle checked, so what else is new? 11–Zebra is out of service, decon and restock, after they opened their night with a messy arrest. So we get sent over to One–O–Five and Columbus Avenue, for an overturned vehicle. It's their area but they're all the way over on Nine–Six and Two, continuing to get their rig back in shape. So Rob tells Central that his unit isn't ready to except an assignment yet, then says to thank the buff boys for taking the job. I liked that title, even though it was sarcasm, and we let Central know we would be responding.

When we get to the scene, it's pretty busy. There are a lot of firemen and cops. The police are talking to two guys who are barely hurt, just a couple of minor cuts and lacerations. And as we walk on over towards an upside-down Suzuki Samurai, our patrol supervisor pulls up to the scene. We go check out the patients, and they both want to RMA. So Brendan and the lieutenant are talking with these guys, and suggesting they go over to St. Luke's, if for nothing else only to get checked out. They don't want to go, and they're really lucky, all things considered. Brendan and I both know they're not hurt bad, but he covers our asses by making a big deal out of refusing medical attention or transport.

I get the paperwork done, and our lieutenant signs off on it. We go back into service, and I tell Brendan, "we're right by the bagel store, come-on, I'll treat you to a coffee." "All right," he says, and we start towards One–Ten and Broadway. So as we're rolling I'm saying, "you know B, if you ever get one of those vehicles, maybe you should just put the license plate on upside down." "I'm not getting one, don't worry," he replied, as he drove right by the bagel store. I asked him "are you a fucking rookie, don't you know where we get coffee?" "No, I'm just not going to watch you eat one of those disgusting fucking fish bagels," he said.

So we went and got Chinese food instead, and I commented "I don't care if I do this a hundred years, I'll never get used to buying my dinner through bullet-proof plexi-glass." So I get pepper steak and onions with fried rice, and B orders a half a dozen chicken wings. When he asks the girl for extra hot sauce, I knew I needed to go out for a second. And I walked a couple of stores down to the bodega, and purchased a pack of Philly blunts.

I went back and paid for my food, and as we were leaving the store, he asked where I went. I told him if he was going to eat the wings with the death sauce, this would be the first time I actually smoked these cigars, without re-rolling them first. We both ate fast, and I was thinking thank God the weather was good, this way when the farting barrage comes, at least I can keep the window open without freezing my nuts off.

We were barely done with our food when Central sends us and 16–David to a cardiac arrest. It's in my favorite complex, 3333 Broadway, and I'm really hating this place, because we can't get the rig into the complex. No matter what building you're going to, you have to walk about a quarter of a mile, with all your shit. So I'm bitching about this, and Brendan calls up the job on the KDT. It clearly states that this is a crime scene, and PD is requesting a crew to come pronounce. It further states that the victim is purple and stiff. But, since we're on a highly intelligent phone-triage system, this is categorized as a cardiac arrest, requiring a dual ALS and BLS response.

Well this is the kind of bullshit we love. It takes you out of service for an hour or so, for nothing. But, if you're one of the other units out there, it sucks, because your going to have to cover your own area and someone else's, and you might not have backup available, since there are now two units out of service, for nothing. Anyway, we get up to a seventeenth floor apartment in D building. It took us fifteen minutes just to get from the rig to the apartment, where we quickly confirm that, yes, this purple-headed, stiff man, laying on a bed next to an empty cash box, and who was strangled with a shoelace from a work boot, was indeed dead. Brendan lit his Macanudo cigar, a fresh one, and I put one of my Phillies to good use. The stink wasn't severe enough for the Vick's, but it was definitely worthy of two cigars. Brendan gave me a light, and I looked over at him and said, "a fresh cigar, this guy should feel honored," and I knew this one would last him all night, and probably into the morning.

I was going to work with a new guy from Met, but the unit wound up getting run down. So I was mandated for a unit that wasn't even running. I was already in the mind set that I was staying, so I asked Sy, who was practically living at the station anyway, if he wanted to get changed, and do some easy BLS overtime. This was cool. By the time all the bureaucracy was cleared up, and we found a vehicle and stocked it, it was already 10 o'clock. I finished my tour after playing car service all night, and in the morning I got mandated.

Jimmy was on the desk, and he wasn't breaking anyone's balls. I thought he was in a good mood, so I figured I would test the water. I asked, "since I was mandated for a minimum of four hours, and my tour was already done since 8, could we be back by 12, and in time for lunch?" He wasn't buying this, as I was instructed "it's the unit that needs to be in service for four hours, not you." So he thanked me for staying, and asked that he not see us again until two o'clock.

So we're cruising around the area, when we get a job for a cardiac arrest. The assignment is in a funeral parlor, up on St. Nicholas Terrace. We get to the scene first, before the medic unit we were backing up. While being led in, we're walking past all these caskets, making some pretty bad jokes about this place, to ourselves. Anyway, there's a small apartment in the back of this parlor, and we find a ninety-two year old woman, in bed. She's unresponsive, and pulseless. We let 13–Willie know that we have an arrest, and keep coming.

We set the woman down on the floor, and begin CPR. Riding BLS, we have a semi-automatic defibrillator, and not a LifePak-12. So we attach it to the patient, and we got a V-fib, as the computer voice is telling us, "shock patient…shock patient." Neither of us noticed the nitro paste on this lady, and no one volunteered to tell us, she was recently prescribed this.

So we clear, and Sy hits the shock button—Foom—this flaming shot of nitro, goes flying off the patient, and burned a hole right into the wall. We both said "Holy Shit," at the same time, then continued to do CPR. We got the patient packaged. As 13–Willie showed up, we were already coming out of the building. We got the patient onto their vehicle, and they ran the ALS part of the arrest, en route to CPMC.

When we were done with the assignment, we were able to laugh about our close call. I said to Sy, "that was really fucked up, and it happened so fast, that I didn't even have time to get scared, or react." And he replied to me, "we were lucky we didn't burn a hole through the patient," because that would have been unexplainable, and we'd be retiring from the academy's retraining program.

We got back in service, and my mind was quickly taken off the subject by our next job. It was pretty quiet, and it was right after 12, as we get an assignment that comes over as an MVA, right over on

One–Three–Six and St. Nick. That's where we were headed anyway, and when we pull up it looks like really minor damage to both cars. We're both thinking allstateitis, as Sy is telling me, "this is real bullshit."

We're getting the bags out of the side door, and a hysterical young woman, covered with blood, is rushing up to the rig screaming, "hurry, hurry, he needs oxygen." So for a split second, I'm thinking that what could be so bad that this lady is so out of control.

As we rush over to the cars, we find in one of them a small six-year-old boy, who had been sitting in the front seat, on his mother's lap. Upon impact, the airbag inflated, and exploded up against the kid's face. Well, he looks like a human Pez dispenser. The boy was a three-quarter decap, and you could see a hole, the size of a baseball, in the front of his throat, as his neck was broken, and head pushed all the way back.

This was completely fucked-up. We transported him down the block to Harlem Hospital, but there was nothing to be done. Anyway, these jobs were the furthest thing, from the easy BLS overtime I thought we would be doing today. We went back to the station, and Jimmy mercifully put us out of service.

I went home, and my uniform wasn't even off, before I was calling the station to bang out that night. This was one day I wasn't going back to start the whole fucking endless process again.

CHAPTER 20

After I banged out, I had a three-day swing. On my days off, I decided I wasn't gonna dwell on misery. I thought, I've got a decent size piece of property, so why don't I enjoy it. I took my daughter over to the nursery and we bought a box of marigolds and a whole load of other plants. I filled up the back of my station wagon and for three days all we did was plant flowers and bushes. Little did I know what a fantastic and productive outlet I had found. Every time I had a fucked up night I would do some gardening during the day. After a while my property started to resemble a home and garden centerfold. As I moved on to planting trees and shrubs, building flower beds and a pond, chopping down old dead trees, and putting up walls made of stones that I found. This job provided me with plenty of aggravation that I could channel into beauty, and this is was the best way I could come up with, to try to get some of my brain cells back.

So when I go back, I'm riding on Victor with Matt. I haven't seen him in a while, and when I find out we're working together, I'm thinking it's gonna be a good night. I'm still feeling fucked up about the kid job. It's got a spot on me right up there with the mother under the Christmas tree. I'm telling myself, deal with it and move on. The problem is, I'm not, and I'm starting to show it. I don't respond well to people I think are fortunate to be clueless as to what's happening out here, and its becoming harder to tolerate people I don't respect professionally telling me how to do things, and what to say. I've figured because you pass a seventy-five question multiple choice test, this doesn't make you my leader, and it certainly doesn't mean you can tell me how it is to do a double shooting at three in the morning up on the fifteenth floor. A lot of people think I have an attitude problem and I do, but it's just a little one. Anyway, I'm really not caring anymore, whose toes I step on, being that my feet have already been crushed. I'm doing this insanity all night long and I'm taking care of my kids all day, one of whom is handicapped and unbelievably demanding, plus I'm commuting almost four hours a day, and a lot of days I'm doing my hours at night and someone else's in the morning. So when I see Matt, I'm trying to be happy. I don't want to start dumping my shit on him, but he's pretty smart and he knows I'm not feeling well tonight.

We get into service and try to get a coffee, but the radio inflicts reality on us. We get sent down to One–Two–Six and Madison for an unconscious seventy-year-old male. When we get up to the apartment, we find this guy out on the floor between the bathroom and the hall. Our patient had recently been prescribed the newest wonder drug, Viagra, which apparently worked beautifully for this guy. His problem started when all his excess energy and activity caused him to have chest pain. So, not thinking anything about it, he started to drop his nitros. I guess his doctor forgot to tell him this could cause irreversible hypotension. So, when Matt does a blood pressure he finds out this guy is fifty palp and pretty unresponsive. I wind up intubating him while Matt is on the phone for orders. When he came back, we started a dopamine drip, but it didn't do anything. We took this patient around the corner to North General and I don't think he ever left.

As we were leaving, Matt told me "at least he went out smiling." I was shocked, I said "Matt you made a funny; I didn't know Vulcan's had a sense of humor," and this time we made sure to get our coffee before we went available. As we're having coffee, I'm talking with Matt about bullshit and responsibilities. I'm saying how I would just like to fuck everything and split, maybe go be a medic in Colorado or something. Matt told me, "wherever you go people are people" and "the bullshit is everywhere." He also said he liked me because I wasn't a bootlicker and that I said what was on my mind, he added that assholes don't like knowing that they're assholes, which is something I loved pointing out.

So I'm thinking this makes me feel a little better as I tell him "you know there's a lot of people working here, that just need to grow a pair of balls and bring their problems on like a man, instead of being a bunch of criticizing, back stabbing, scumbags." I also mentioned, I was through being nice to hypocrites. I told him I would punch someone in the face but I would never stab them in the back, as the radio broke my chain of thought. It told us One–Sixteen and Riverside Drive for difficulty breathing. A twenty-four year old female asthmatic.

When we pulled up to the scene, this guy was already in the lobby with a girl, who was working very hard to get her breath. We carried her right into the rig, where we quickly saw she was completely closed off. She was panicked and I realized on this job that the crashing asthmatic is the hardest tube I would ever do. We put her on the stretcher and I tried to bag her as Matt got on the telemetry unit for medical control orders. I attempted to push some air into the frantic patient with the BVM, as she flailed away. I got a 7.5 ET tube set up while trying my best to keep this girl on the stretcher. The doc on the other end could hear the commotion in the background and he quickly gave Matt the orders we needed. Matt drew up and gave .3 of Epi sub Q as I went in her with a Mac3. Well this girl didn't give a shit, we were trying to save her life. All she knew was she couldn't breathe, and I was sticking this long metal curved blade down her throat. As I put the Laryngoscope in her mouth, her arm came up and hit me right in the face. I saw stars for a second and I felt the blood run out of my nose and onto her face and hair. I put my right forearm on her forehead and held the tube with that hand. I went in quickly with the left hand and saw the closed off vocal chords for a split second, as I banged the tube right through them. I knew it was good, but there was still a lot of resistance as I tried to breath for her. I dumped a provental down the tube and bagged her like crazy. Matt hit a line and pushed 125 milligrams of solumedrol. I started to bag, as our patient tried to inhale. The resistance lessened and I went from about forty-eight a minute down to twenty-four. We jetted over to St. Luke's and they knew we were coming. When we were getting the ACR signed, the nurse said we did great, and gave me a cold pack for my swollen face, cause by this time I was covered in blood and definitely needed to change my shirt.

We go back to the station and I get myself cleaned up while Matt gets us restocked, I still had over five hours left in my tour and I already felt like I was ready to leave for the day. We were cruising the neighborhood, and I was watching the local artists putting up some new murals on store fronts, unless they had permission, working under the late night street lights was the safest way to paint without being arrested. Anyway, I was thinking this guy was really good, as I watched him do a religious scene, on a maroon brick wall.

Well we hear 11–Zebra and 12–Bravo get a job in the subway, on One–Ten and Broadway for a traumatic arrest. We can hear on the PD radio that they got a guy under the train. So Matt knows I'm dying to check this out. We cruise over on an available basis, to see if we can buff any of this. By the time we got there ESU was getting ready to get this guy out from under the train. He was an obvious DOA, who witnesses said, looked drunk and apparently he jumped down onto the tracks, on the local side. He walked down to the end of the tunnel, and started to take a shit on the tracks, right at the far end of the platform. By the time he knew a train was coming his drawers were still down around his ankles, and he had no chance to climb back up. The train sped into the station, splattering this guy's head all over the tracks. The whole top and back of his skull was gone and there was shit and brain matter covering this guy. We had to leave the scene, because there were captains, lieutenants, and chiefs all over the place and we were getting a job of our own. As we headed up the concrete stairs to the street, I said to Matt, "that asshole gave new meaning to the phrase shit for brains, didn't he?" and I could see Matt was back to normal, because I didn't even get a response from him.

So we get sent all the way up to One–Six–Four and Amsterdam, for an OB complication. Sure enough, this was a complete waste of 911 resources. We climb up five flights of stairs, and find a young overweight, Spanish woman, who's in labor. Her contractions are about six minutes apart, and she's got plenty of time, I thought. So she's got a little suitcase packed and we figure, all right let's do the taxi thing, four blocks over to CPMC. But no, the husband tells us she's gotta go to Roosevelt Hospital all the way down on Fifty-ninth Street. To top it off he's already spoken to telemetry via his 911 call, and this transport has been pre-approved, before we even have to call a patrol supervisor. Not only that, no one was exactly running to help us carry her. She had no intention of walking as she's doing her impersonation of Roseanne on Qualudes. But, I already know we ain't carrying her, I tell the husband, just to be safe he needs to help Matt and I carry her. This was all he needed to hear, as he spoke to her in Spanish, all of a sudden a miracle occurred, and her mental status immediately improved, enough for her to walk the five flights for us. This job took us out of service for over an hour and a half, since we had to bring her up to the labor delivery room and neither of us had any idea where it was.

We snuck back uptown, and tried to hide out up on Broadway and One–Two–Eight. We actually both fell out for about an hour, and the sun was soon gonna be up. All I needed now was to get mandated I thought, as the person on the other end of the radio figured, as long as I'm up getting my donuts, why don't I give 16–Victor a bullshit job.

We get sent over to One–Five–Six and Amsterdam for an unconscious on the street. We find a really obnoxious drunk, who's pissed, because I won't let him sleep in the street up against the curb. So we pick him up by his belt loops and put him on the stretcher. He's covered in puke and piss and now I've just about had enough. I'm telling Matt, "you see what I mean, it never fucking ends." "I gotta be on top of my game for this scumbag all night long, then I'm so physically exhausted all day, I'm skelling out on my own kids." So this guy is really pissing me off, and he spits on me as I'm trying to do a blood pressure. I tell Matt "who knows, maybe he fell, and that's why he's laying up against the curb." "I think he needs to be immobilized on the long board." So Matt didn't exactly know what I was doing, but being the sharp guy that he is, he figured it best to humor me. So I lay down the head of the stretcher and slide the orange long board under this guy. We tie his hands to the side and his feet to the bottom. As I slide a nice tight no neck collar around him, he tries to spit on me again, but this time I'm ready. I stuffed a six-inch roll of cling in his mouth, then taped a non-rebreather over it with that thick super stick two-inch tape. Our boy was getting plenty of air, and was in no danger. So when I secured his head to the board, I took the same roll of tape and went right across his big bushy eyebrows with it. When we got to the ER, I removed the cling before we pulled in. I presented him to the triage nurse as a non-English speaking intox, fall victim. He was flailing pretty good and giving the nurses a lot of trouble too. The doctor quickly ascertained, that Hector didn't need to be on the board, and told us we could take it back. This is just what I wanted. I cut the cravats that secured his arms and legs, and then with a quick rip, I gave this schmuck instant electrolysis. Removing all of his eyebrows, and probably some skin, while taking the tape off his forehead. This got him really agitated, so security pig piled him and four pointed him to the bed.

So when we're thinking that we can go back for the change, they squeeze one more out of us at One–Four–Eight, between Broadway and Amsterdam for a jumper down. We get there fast and we have a BLS backup, it's Alex and Joey, and they're just getting their day started with this job as we're ending ours. We get to the address and we're told the guy is behind the building and that he's pretty messed up. We get led through a basement apartment and out into a yard. It's the only was to get out there, and it hasn't been cleaned in years. The weeds are three feet tall and garbage has had plenty of time to accumulate and stagnate. On top of that, it's a minefield of dog shit. So there's a few cops over there and a middle aged Spanish man speaking to them. He's the guy who made the call, when he saw out his bathroom window, this guy lying out there in the yard. So the cops are trying to get their tour over too, they're not into extra paperwork. We tell them, ok he was an attempted suicide not a burglar, but the reality was this guy was trying to break into the top floor apartment through the window, from the roof, when he found out he really wasn't Spiderman. So Matt and I are talking to the guy with the cops, he's speaking really fast and is very descriptive with his hands. I ask, "how long has he been down here?" So our witness starts telling us, "you know I was drinking last night, so I'm in the shower and out of my corner of my eye I think I see him fly by my window, but then I think, hey man, you know I'm still fucked up, no one is flying." So I finish my shower and when I look out my window, I think oh my god, there's this guy out there. So I call you, and you come. I looked back at Matt and I said, "about twenty minutes." By this time, the cops are convinced he's a jumper and not a robber, so there's minimal paper work and no arrest. I tell them get home safe and I'm saying to Alex at least they're getting off on time, as they take a fifty-five from us and leave the scene.

Matt drops a fourteen in one arm and I hit one in the other. This guy is awake and alert but he ain't answering any questions. We cut his clothes off and get his information from his wallet. We put him in the BLS rig and I rode with Alex, as Matt and Joey drove our units over to Harlem. We banged this job out relatively quickly and we only got an hour of unwanted overtime.

When we got back to the station, Matt got mandated and he was gonna have to work with Brendan, who was also getting mandated, but today I wasn't up and I got to go home. When I was cruising over the

George Washington Bridge, I slipped in a Pearl Jam tape and lit up. I cruised all the way up to exit nine before I put my bone out which by this time was el' roacho. I thought I'm lucky I wasn't up to get mandated today cause I would have told lieutenant lard ass to lick my nuts, before I would have done six more hours. When I got home I planted a row of hostas and a Japanese red maple tree. I got a little sleep, and then went back to start the whole fucking endless process again.

CHAPTER 21

The last few days the weather has been really hot. Fortunately it's not so bad on the overnights. Summer is in full effect, and everyone seems to stay out late. I've noticed that the streets are busier at 3:30 a.m. than they are at 7:30. I've been working 6–Victor with Jason and things are good for us. The unit is staying busy, and more important, it's staying in service. So we start our night like any other. Sign our drugs out and get a job, before the rig is even checked.

We're sent over to One–Two–Five and the FDR, for an MVA, with injuries. On the scene there's already plenty of firemen and cops. We got an overturned BMW that also took down a light-post. There are two young white girls, about 20 and 22, talking to the cops, and trying to bullshit their way out of some drug paraphernalia that was found in the car. Apparently these kids came over from Jersey to cop some dope, and the police are giving them a hard time, and telling the young ladies if any drugs are found, they are going to be arrested. They're swearing up and down they don't have any drugs, and since they are in the southbound lane, I'm telling Jason "yeah, because they didn't get any yet." So we ask them if they're all right, and they come into the rig to get checked out. Both girls are pretty much fine, and this is the thing about overturns, there is no middle ground. Either you're barely scratched, or a DOA. So one girl is whining that her hand hurts, and nothing else. The other has slight back pain, and I guess she figures going to the hospital will get the cops off her case. So I'm listening to these chicks bitching about how the cops have some nerve harassing them. Finally I can't take anymore. I say to one of them, "listen sweetheart you just don't get it, do you?" "You should be thanking God you're not on page 3 of tomorrows Daily News." "And your parents are lucky the cops are not on the phone with them right now, telling them he's sorry to inform them that you were killed in a car crash." So now they're feeling pretty small, since they realize they are not getting any sympathy from us. I immobilized the one who was saying her back hurt, being extra careful not to mess up her hair, of course. And I gave the other a cold pack for her hand. We then took our unchecked vehicle down to Met, and dropped them off, so they could call daddy from the hospital and get some real sympathy.

After the job, I suggested that we get some of that nuclear barrio coffee, and I came back with three cups. Jason asked who the third one was for, and I said "me," as I poured both of them into one big cup, and gave him the other. I already knew I was next up on the mandate list, and I continued, "I'm going to need plenty of caffeine and nicotine to get through the next twelve hours. So we're cruising back up to our area along Second Avenue, and the barrio is busy. There's people hanging out on every corner, and me and Jason are just bullshitting about baseball, as we pass through. He lives in Queens, so he roots for the Mets. I like the Bombers. Anyway, my team had just taken three straight from his, and I got the last word.

We got hit with a sick job on One–Three–Eight and Five. This is right around the corner from the hospital. By now I've learned a sick job could be a cardiac arrest, or an arrest can end up being a little old man holding a suitcase, needing a ride to the clinic. It's a roll of the dice every job. So the text is showing 12-year-old male has muscle aches, and is in pain. Well even the most optimistic person would think this has bullshit job written all over it. We had to walk up to the fourth floor, because it was recently confirmed that Station 18 personnel were only allowed to have patients that got sick above three flights up. I mentioned the last time I had a ground floor sick job, was during the Bush administration, and my partner agreed saying, "for some great unknown mystery of man, you never get a sick job down low, unless it's in the subway." When we get to the apartment, we got serious real fast. We found a kid who was in agony. He had sickle cell anemia, and this was the first time I had witnessed this. He was in so much pain, we couldn't even touch him without him screaming out. I felt horrible that I couldn't do anything to help this child. It was really heartbreaking hearing his cries, as we packaged and carried him down to the unit. I did everything I could to help him not hurt, but I was very happy it was only a thirty-second ride to the hospital. When we went back in service, I told my partner, "these jobs fuck me up as much as the shootings," and he agreed, saying that job was gut-wrenching. I sincerely wished I was smarter, so I could do something about all this fucking disease and misery.

As soon as we go available, we get another assignment—One–Five–Eight and Douglas, for an anaphylactic reaction. Now this job was bullshit, no two ways about it. The KDT is stating 27-year-old male with a rash on his genitalia. So how much does this suck, we still don't even have our vehicle fully checked. We get sent to a complex that has the same address on sixteen different entrances, labeled A through P. But of course we don't have a letter to find this asshole, whose allegedly experiencing an anaphylactic reaction, which is nothing more than a summertime heat rash, on his balls. So we finally find the right building. I don't even need to say he was on the fifth floor, which is actually 10 of those winding flights. So this guy is pretty cranky. He's in an empty apartment, except for an old couch and a mattress. It's like two hundred degrees in here, and his balls are on fire. The patient tells us he's been using Benadryl, but it's not helping. So I'm thinking the hospital is looking real good to this guy. He shuffles down to the bus, and we take him over to Harlem. In the emergency room, Jason tells the nurse with a straight face, that our patient is experiencing an allergic reaction to sweat, on his critical one-percent. And as we're walking out, I said "see, that's why I let you do the talking."

So we're hanging out by the ER bay. I see Sy, and we start to bullshit a little. I'm busting his chops that he needs to barbecue again soon. And maybe we can use some nitro paste to get the coal started. I had told Jason about our nitro shrapnel incident, and he got a kick out of the way Sy re-told the story. So we're telling him about this guy with the rotten crotch, and I'm thinking what a pain in the ass people can be. But I had no idea, what the next job would bring.

We get an assignment on One–Four–Five and Amsterdam for an OB comp. We arrive at a dirty, cramped, dark apartment, to find a twenty-six year old, full-term, pregnant crack-head. The woman said her water broke this morning and she started hitting the pipe, as soon as she went into labor. So she's been smoking crack for seventeen hours now, and she's nuts. Her contractions were about two minutes apart, and some-one in the room with her called the ambulance. She's telling us she doesn't want this baby, and she's not going to let it be born. This woman is completely irrational, and I tell Jason "this is a bad time to decide you don't want the baby." So we request a PD unit to the scene, and also a backup. At this point the woman is saying to us, as the baby pops out, she's going to squeeze its head with her knees and kill it. I pull Jason to the side, and I tell him "I'm not fucking around with this lunatic, try to keep her calm, while I call medical control and get a discretionary order for valium." When I get off the phone, 13–Charlie and the cops arrive to help. Ziffy was working with Manny-crime-scene, who got mandated for overtime, and really wasn't in the mood for this craziness either. Anyway, Jason had this woman somewhat calm, but when the police and EMT's come in she starts geekin' again, screaming and slapping at us. We get her tied into the stair chair, and her contractions are about a minute apart. I say to Zif, "we're not delivering this one." "Jason's hitting a line, we're knocking her out, then we're jettin to CPMC." I ask Jason, "please don't miss," and like the champ that he is, he banged an 18 right below her elbow. We wound up pushing 20 mg of Valium, then notified Columbia that we were coming. It was a straight run up Amsterdam, about 45 seconds.

We got into the emergency room, and I was happy to be done with her. We were out of service for a while restocking the narcotics, and there was minimal mess on the rig. So the job was a success after all, but I couldn't help feeling nothing but sorrow for the future of that baby. I was feeling pretty burnt already, and I still had like 8 more hours to go.

I couldn't believe the ignorance, immaturity and irresponsibility that I constantly encountered. During my life a lot of people had really made me feel like a worthless fuck-up. But I knew I wasn't and I really was starting to see that I was a good man, just trying really hard to do right. I figured out on this night that was the key, a lot of people don't even try. I'm really tired, but I'm feeling all right when the onslaught continues. The mandate comes down, and I know I'll be staying until the after-noon. So Jason asks the Lieutenant if another vacancy opens up, let him know, and he'll just stay with me and roll the unit over. This was really cool, because the next person up to get mandated would have been Tom, and he's not exactly the most fun guy to be around after he's been ordered to stay around for someone else's hours. So midnight turns into morning. Insanity has come to be the norm, and the radio voice of doom plays its favorite tune. "6–Victor, 3–David, One–Twelve and Riverside for the arrest." Just what we needed I thought, a wake up dead. Early morning arrests are almost always real, but this one was different.

We get to one of those single-room occupancy welfare buildings, and the whole place smells like bad feet. So I guess strange odors coming out of doors just goes unnoticed. The manager of this place had finally decided he had to get into a room up there, because no one saw the resident in a while, and they didn't know if he was even still there. So before we even get to the door, I'm lighting a stinky Macanudo and grabbing the jar of Vicks that I now always carry, thanks to Brendan. Jason has his own

Vicks, and even though he doesn't smoke, felt a need to puff a cigar. The manager tells us this is really bad, as he puts a red bandana over his face, and we gob up the Vicks gel under our noses. When the door opens, we see this decomposed corpse on the bed. He's been like this so long, it looks like he's burned up. He's almost a skeleton already. "Holy Shit," Jason says, "even the maggots wouldn't go near this." The oozing body fluid had made a thick hard stain all over the mattress and floor, that made your feet stick like flypaper. And we figured if we had gotten this job six months ago, this guy still would have been decomposed. We tell the manager, we'll get PD, to have the body, or what's left of it, removed.

We went back down to the rig to finish the paperwork for the night. As I thumbed through the ACR's, I thought about another night spent on the plantation. Let's see what the rest of the morning brings. So we go back to the station and roll out for tour two. Since Jason had volunteered for the overtime, we only had to keep the unit in service for four hours. So even thought I was mandated for six, in reality, if everything went well, I could be out of there by twelve o'clock. We were parked over by St. Nick park, on One–Three–Eight. I was enjoying a steak and egg sandwich, while Jason was reading. We were both completely exhausted, but it was one of those few times I actually wanted a job, because it would wake me up a little, and the time would go faster. So I finish eating, which was a minor miracle in itself. It's almost nine thirty, and we still haven't had a morning job yet. I looked over at Jason, as I lit a cigarette, and asked, "what is the city broken or something, it's too calm out here." He responded that I had just put a curse on us, but the radio remained silent.

A little before 10, we got hit. "One–Four–Four, and Lenox, for the jumper down." We're backing up 13–David. They get to the scene first, and it was Alex and Joey. I hear Alex ask us for an ETA, as he calls traumatic arrest. I let him know we're less than 30 seconds away, as we fly down One–Four–Five. When we get there, we have a twenty-five year old female, who jumped off the roof of the building, thirty floors above. She went right through the top of a tree, and was lying in the courtyard, between the building and the walking path. She should have been an 83, and left with PD, but she was clearly in public view, and there was already a big crowd gathered around her, expecting us to do something. Alex came back with the long board, and a collar, and I said to Joey, "it's Nike time, just do it," as we log rolled her onto the board, and collared her. I could tell immediately that her neck and jaw were broken, as I tubed her right there on the sidewalk. Thirty seconds later, we were in the rig, and Jason was dropping a fourteen in her as Alex cut her clothes off. When her blood stained sweatpants came off, it looked like she was wearing red underwear, from all the blood. Alex cut them off too, and we saw that she had been vaginally split, like a wishbone, as a result of slamming down onto a thick tree branch, right before hitting the concrete. Once inside the rig, we all knew there was no way in hell this woman would survive. The only question was, was it suicide or murder? Which we weren't really able to help the detectives with.

By the time we finished the clean up and restock, its 11:30. This was bad timing, because there was no way we could skate another half-hour without getting another job. So my plan of heading up the Palisades by 12, went up in smoke, about as fast as this woman's life had blinked out. About 10 to 12, we get the inevitable late-job.

We're sent up to One–Two–Five and B'way, for the ped struck. As we arrive, we find a Chinese food delivery boy, who had been on his bike, and hit by a bus. He wasn't dead, but he was really fucked-up. The bike was mangled, and halfway under the bus, but our patient was just a little bit luckier. He had a broken leg that got spun around backwards, right below the knee. And he had some really nasty facial abrasions. One of which had scraped off a good part of his mustache. So we get him on the board and in the rig. I dropped a line, as Jason splinted him. When we went en route, I cleaned up his road-rash with some sterile saline, and we were out of the ER by 12:40, which wasn't too bad. I took an easy cruise up the Palisades in the right lane, and was home before 2:30. I actually got a few hours sleep, and still had time to shit, shower and shave, before I went back to start the whole fucking endless process again.

CHAPTER 22

So, Jason and I are out here tearing things up. We back up everyone without question, even if we know they're dicks. We had been kicking so much ass, when I came to the station tonight there was a very complimentary cartoon circulating featuring us as the ninja medics. We had a really good laugh over this as we got the unit in service.

There was a new guy at the station, Richie B, from the Bronx. He was sent to work overnights in Harlem by the bureaucrats at headquarters as punishment for having a pair of balls and not taking any shit from supervisors out there. So as we were leaving the station, we were introduced to him by Sy. Like myself, Richie was very abrasive and although we didn't like each other at first, I knew he lived by his own misunderstood code of honor and I respected him. Richie had a lot of years under his belt in the South Bronx and another thing that I liked about him was he didn't hold a signal and lie, he would back up anyone. So as part of his punishment, he's breaking in a quiet, frail rookie, I call Junior. A lot of people at the station have been fucking with Junior and I knew Richie felt like he was alone on an Island, when he had to work with him. Anyway, I liked Junior. I saw he had potential and I would give him a vote of confidence now and then. So me, Jason and Brendan would back them up a lot, and vice versa and we established a real good working relationship.

So we get a job up near 3333 Broadway, and by now you're probably as tired of this address as we were, it's for an altered mental status. When we get to the building across the street from this complex, some guy meets us out front and tells us his neighbor was acting weird and walking the hallway naked. So we get to the hall and by this time, the guy was back in his apartment. We knock on the door and yes, a naked man about six-foot three, two hundred and seventy pounds, opens up. He tells us to come in. So we take about two steps into the apartment and the door closes behind us. Right away you can tell this guy is high as a kite. He's really babbling to himself as he's walking around a large dinning room table quickly. When we try to talk to him he's getting really agitated. We go to step out of the apartment, but the doorknob is fucked up and when Jason goes to turn it, it falls off onto the floor. So he's telling me, "this is not good," and we can't get the door open. I come up on the air and I ask Central if we can get PD to the scene. The dispatcher says, "ten-four I'll put in the request," then says, "6–Victor are you in any danger at this time?" Well this guy is getting really paranoid about the radio, so I ask Central "can we just get a unit here forthwith," and I left it keyed up so they could hear this maniac.

Well it turns out this guy had been speedballing with coke and a brand of heroin called polo. This stuff was real nasty, and cut with schapolamine. So our patient ain't lettin' us near him, we're doing a pretty good job of keeping our distance, and I turned down the radio that was freaking him out. Well anyway, 11–Zebra and 16–David arrived, before the cops even got there. I had only met Richie a few minutes ago, but he was already putting his ass on the line for us, and Zebra had a big time reputation as an excellent unit that we highly respected. We were glad to see the four of them come into the apartment, as they had no problem getting the door open from the outside. They immediately see our problem and the six of us stepped out into the hall to wait for PD.

Well when the cops get there, at first he wouldn't answer the door. All he had to do was put a pair of pants on and act semi rational and we all would have went away. But no, this guy comes out of the apartment completely naked and completely irrational and he's really lucky he didn't have a knife or anything, cause they would have blown his head off. So now he's out in the hall again and he's acting more like an anticholenergic overdose and not heroin. Anyway it becomes apparent that he needs to be restrained and escorted to psych. We get the stretcher in the hall and it takes four cops to get him on it, so we can get him tied down. We ran AMS on him but the cocktail was ineffective. In the emergency room they gave him more narcan and he started having a seizure. They knocked him out then he got intubated and our night was off and running in typical fashion.

So our next job, we get sent around to One–Four–Three and Powell for a cardiac arrest. Ziffy and Derek are backing us up. We get to the building and it's the same old story. The smell of piss in the elevator alleviates the smell of crack in the lobby. We get to the apartment and we have a thirty-two year old female who has advanced cancer. The woman is not in arrest but she's kind of lethargic for someone who is awake and oriented. This woman is about sixty pounds and there was nothing more the hospital could do for her. So she had been discharged, basically to die with dignity in her home, with her family and not in the hospital. Well the husband had been doubling, tripling and quadrupling her morphine doses, because of the unbearable pain she was in. He told us he thought she had stopped breathing. Well you could see the effects her condition was having on him. He was extremely anxiety stricken and very sad. He told us, all her records were at Mount Sinai and that's where she was being treated. So this patient is breathing well on her own and although her blood pressure is 90/60 base line, the four of us decide that we'll take her and Ziffy and Derek can eighty-seven and get something to eat. Jason and I put her in the stair chair and made her as comfortable as possible. Being that the slightest movement caused severe pain, this was difficult at best. We got down to the unit, and I let the husband ride in the back with us, as we went to Mount Sinai.

Well a couple of days later, I got in a lot of trouble because I didn't give her two milligrams of narcan, which would have intensified all her pain and probably made her vomit. I didn't lay her down flat on a stiff aluminum scoop stretcher, and I didn't take her to the nearest 911 receiving hospital. A hospital she had never been in and knew nothing about her history. So I knew I did nothing wrong. I told the captain "if this is the way it is, then maybe I don't belong here." Well I ate a three-day restriction, and was becoming known as a loose cannon with the bureaucrats and politicians at the station. Sy had warned me about these blowjobs, but since I didn't respect them I really didn't give a shit.

So the rest of the night goes fairly easy. We do a real asthma and a real MI (heart attack). Things slow down before sunrise and we go park by the water so we can nod out a little. I hear the radio send 13–Willie to the polo grounds for an arrest and about a half-hour later, the radio wakes me up, as I hear Brendan asking dispatch to give a notification for him. So I'm awake now and I'm watching the sunrise over the George Washington Bridge, above the Hudson River and I'm feeling really relaxed. About 7:15, just as I was beginning to think we could possibly get off on time tonight, we get hit. "6–Victor," a tired voice calls out. I pick up the mic and I groan back, "Victor go." "One–Four–Seven and Amsterdam for the cardiac arrest." "6–David on the back." So we head over and Jason tells me he's not up for working an arrest now, and I came back with, "yeah I got nothing better to do either, so lets go see who thought this would be a good morning to die."

We arrive in front of a store as PD is waiting to get in. It's one of these religious Santeria shops or something. Well you can see in the window and there's a body in there. A real innocent looking old lady opens the door and lets us all in. We get close to the stiff cold, purple body, lying on an old hardwood floor with a lot of sawdust, next to a glass counter. There were about forty or fifty candles burning around him and there were a couple of chickens and a rooster walking around. Well this guy was completely rigored out as Jason calmly asked, "Ma'am, how long has he been like this?" She just looked at him blankly and didn't say anything. By the length of the candles it was pretty clear this set up was done last night and I whispered to Junior, "I guess the chickens aren't working." I figured this was a cultural thing and I didn't want to seem completely insensitive, so I kept my mouth shut. I let Jason do the talking and we made this job an eighty-three left with PD, and I actually did get off on time, as there was only minor paperwork to do on this job.

So I meet Sy outside the station and we go over to One–Three–Two and Lenox for breakfast. I'm always starvin' after work and this was the best way to calm down a little. Besides, I knew I was gonna have to mow my lawn today and this was gonna take three or four hours. It was starting to look pretty shaggy as I had been putting this off a couple of weeks by doing planting and pruning. I wanted to stay awake this morning so I could get it done in the early afternoon.

While we eat, we're discussing everything from the Yankees to which female in the station has the best ass. We get to talking about the job and he's telling me one he did on tour three this week with Manny-crime-scene. They get a sick job over on One–Four–Nine and Douglas where they got a little old lady laying on a carpet, and I'm thinking this story is starting innocent enough. Then, Sy goes on to say, she's got cellulitis in her feet that's so bad its oozing and has maggots in the open wounds. "Great," I tell him as I take a sip of coffee. "No, no, it gets better," he says. She looks like she's been laying there about two weeks, her eyes are completely crusted over about a half inch thick and he tells me, they think they got a DOA. So he asks the son, "how long has she been there?" And he confirms she fell about two weeks ago. So Sy asks, "yeah, well why didn't you call us two weeks ago?" And the guy answered because she said she was OK and to just let her lie there. So Manny asked him, "well when was the last time you spoke to her?" And the guy answered, "five minutes before you came." So, I'm dippin' my toast in my coffee and I said, "what are you kidding me?" Sy tells me that he plays along with this guy and he leans over what he thinks is a corpse and asks, "Ma'am, speak to me." Well she answered him saying, "yes dear, what would you like?" They were completely freaked out, the guy told them she didn't want to get up and he had been feeding her, when she asked him to. Today she finally wanted to get up, but was not able to because she was stuck to the rug from lying there so long, in her own body fluids.

Well by now Sy's requested medics and a patrol supervisor for this. They try to get the rug out from under her, but by tearing the rug away they're also tearing her skin off. So he decides they'll cut the rug around her body and transport her on the rug. All the medic units in the area are tied up and the Lieutenant who arrives agrees with Sy, that they shouldn't wait around, and treat the rug as if it were an impaled object, as it would have caused much harm trying to remove it. They wound up transporting to Harlem Hospital and asked the dispatcher to give a notification. Central wanted a set of vitals, but he said they we're unable to obtain them and the emergency room staff would understand when they got there. The patient needed to soak in warm water to get the cement like crust separated away from her. No one in the emergency room had ever seen anything like this, and they were genuinely shocked. Eventually she would wind up being discharged to a nursing home if she were able to recover.

I took an easy ride home, and changed to work in the yard. It took till after two o'clock to get done and halfway through I needed to put together a small pool for my girls. I thought I was gonna melt under the sun out there today. When I got to sleep that afternoon, I was out cold. I woke up at eleven o'clock and I was so fuzzy I didn't know if it was eleven in the morning or eleven at night. Either way, I was in trouble. I got my bearings and saw it was still dark out. I was dressed and out the door in fifteen minutes. I still wasn't fully awake when I got to work, but I was only about forty-five minutes late, which wasn't too bad. And as soon as I got there we were in service as Jason had the rig ready to go.

We had a pretty easy night, all things considered. We didn't get a real job until six in the morning. We had missed a good one about four in the morning because we were transporting a constipated old lady. Brendan was working with Tom on 13–Willie; they had a job for a twenty-five year old guy who hung himself from a tree in St. Nick Park. This would've been our job if we were available, but that was the luck of the draw. And I was told he was a good DOA.

At six in the morning, we got hit for a wake up dead in the colonial park houses. This guy had gone down with an inbleed that was so fucked up he was literally puking chunks of shit. Some of which had dried over his face and looked like a mask of death. He was still warm, and we had to work him. So I use my classic, I'm here cause I love my kids, what's your excuse line, as I kneel down around the shitty vomit and blood. I get this guy tubed and Jason hit a line quick, he dumped an epi and atropine in and we decided to work on the fly and get the fuck off this scene that stunk like a cesspool.

When we got to CPMC the arrest was called pretty quickly and the guy's mouth still had chunky shifty vomit in it. The doctor gave me big time props, asking if I did the tube digitally, saying it was excellent that I could get visualization of the vocal chords. We went back to the station BBP and restock. We were done at seven forty-five and when we got a late job, Brendan picked it up for us. This worked out well cause Brendan and Tom were finishing at nine, and this would take them right up to the change. I got off on time for the second night in a row, this really was rare and I was grateful for this.

CHAPTER 23

Jason's got some pass days and Rod has taken a leave of absence. He had been talking about taking a nursing job that paid more and we don't expect him to come back, especially since he told the captain to kiss his hairy ass before he left. So I'm out here piloting the Starship Victor with Matt tonight. Brendan is in service already with Tom and Matt and I are in service and parked up on the triangle. It's a hot weekend night and I could see it was already busy, just by driving my car the three blocks from the FDR to the parking lot.

So we got sent over to One–Two–Eight and St. Nick for an asthma. We're only thirty seconds from this scene and when we arrive, we get a thirty-six year old male who's wheezing and pretty tight. He's already on the stoop and he meets the unit out front. He's sitting in the rig and I'm letting him hit an alupent treatment while we do his vitals and get information He tells me it's helping, so we give it a second and start to transport him over to St. Luke's. While we're en route, 13–Willie is getting sent to a cardiac arrest with 13–Charlie. It's up on One–Five–Five and the Henry Hudson Parkway. So when we get to St. Luke's, I'm asking Matt what he thinks they got. Being that we can't call up details from their job on our KDT, we're thinking maybe a traumatic arrest, MVA on the parkway. Anyway, my curiosity is peaked and we get out of the emergency room quick. I let Central know we're available and then Ziffy comes up on the air and tells me to go to 10 George, a radio frequency we can speak on, one to one. He says to go back to our area via the parkway and stop over at his scene. I mentioned we didn't want to step on

Tom or Brendan's toes and he said, "Brendan is the one who wanted us to come by." So we head over to their job and it turns out to be a DOA crime scene. Someone really had a good sense of humor in regard to how they sent their message out. They had a guy who was a known drug dealer, executed. He had been shot twice in the back of the head, behind his ear, then whoever did this rolled him up in a rug and dumped him underneath a huge billboard that had a cartoon of McGruff the crime dog and it said, "take a bite out of crime." We were all amused with the vigilante street justice and even the detective's thought it was original. Unfortunately it wasn't gonna stop them from investigating a clear-cut case of murder.

We hung out for a little while till Central catches up with us. We get an assignment for an altered mental status down on One–Two–Six and Five. We get down there to find a woman in her twenties, who's really withdrawn from poverty and drug use. She's not talking much to us but we do find out she's on cogentin and buspar which are two psych drugs. So she's sitting on the curb and has these really strange facial gestures and contorted muscle spasms. It's almost like in between a seizure and Turret's syndrome. So she hasn't had her meds in a few days, and Matt tells me we have something called a dystonic reaction, a sort of withdrawal from the prescribed medications. Anyway, we get her onto the rig and I start an IV. We don't have a protocol for this. The coma cocktail would have done nothing and Matt tells me we need a discretionary order for Benadryl. So we speak to medical control via the telemetry unit and get the order for fifty milligrams slow IV push. This helped our patient a lot and we transported her over to North General without a problem.

We went down into the Barrio to eat and I got a burrito as big as a football. I knew I would be eating this monster all night, so it wasn't much of a bother when Central bellowed for the next assignment. We get sent over to One–Four–O and Lenox for an unconscious on the street. Right away, we think its Levi, but the thing about it is Levi always comes over as a seizure. So we cruise over thinking if it's not Levi then it could be one of about any fifty people who hang out in that park all night. So we get to the scene and low and behold there's no one requiring treatment. Not even Levi. We get out of the rig and walk around the park a little, no one called the unit and aside from the usual, no one looks unconscious. We decide to circle around the block once before we make this a ninety (no patient). As we come off Powell onto One–Four–O again, we get flagged by this girl. We find a guy in between two parked cars near the corner. So this caller really fucked up cause we were really far up from Lenox. Anyway he's out cold and we quickly see that he's in arrest. It turns out the girl was getting high with this guy and she knew nothing about him, not even his name. She said he went between the cars and started to vomit, then he dropped. So we get him in the rig and he's in V-fib. We shock him three times and then I intubate him while Matt gets a line. We give him lidocaine and epi and wound up shocking him like six more times; he never converted from V-fib. I gave bretylliun and more lidocaine. We gave more epi and narcan too. Nothing broke this guy. I think we shocked him about ten times and he stayed fib all the way into the emergency room. He died in the hospital and when we were done, we thought about how burned we would have gotten if we had made him a ninety, because some junkie didn't know she was on Seventh and not Sixth Avenue. So, we were lucky we were on our toes tonight to this point, but the next job really took me off my game.

The radio calls again, "6–Victor." "Victor go," I answered. "One–Eighteen and Three for the burn." So back down into the barrio we go. 12–Young is stuck on an MVA with injuries so we get the job right in the center of their area. Its in apartment 4R, which means rear, as there are only two apartments on each floor—front and rear. Anyway, we step off the rig and from the curb, I can hear a kid crying. I tell Matt this is gonna be bad. I can hear her crying already. So he responds, "you're too negative, think positive." I said, "no, I can really hear her crying, can't you?" But he couldn't, not yet at least. So when we step into the lobby now, you can clearly hear the screams of a child. As we hurry up the winding stairs, the screams intensify until we're in the apartment; at this point they're deafening. This was one of those jobs that really pisses you off. The patient was a four-year-old girl, who had been sick for a couple of days. She was crying most of the night. Her mother couldn't take it any more, and gave this kid a bath in scalding hot water. This kid was screaming at the top of her lungs as we tried to approach her. Her entire vaginal area and buttocks were one huge blister surrounded by a red area, around her lower back and thighs. Well we really couldn't do much on this scene. The mother was arrested, and we transported the little girl over to Harlem Hospital. Both of us were extremely stressed out. By the time we got to the emergency room, even the nurses were horrified and the doctor needed to give her Valium, shortly after our arrival as this kid never stopped screaming except in between breaths. We were out of service about an hour filling out child abuse reports, but it wasn't enough. My head felt like it had a steel wedge going through my temple. Matt wasn't doing much better as he was popping aspirins like tiny tarts.

So night turns into morning, and I find out I'm getting mandated. I'm not happy about it, and I'm really bitchin' up a storm. It doesn't matter though, cause I'm gonna stay or I'm gonna eat a three day pay hit. So at least Matt is going home on time, but not before we get another cardiac arrest. I'm actually hoping for an eighty-three, cause I'm so pissed I can't even think straight, let alone work an arrest. Well fate didn't disappoint me. We go into another of the vertical urinals up into a dirty project apartment. We found yet another DOA that was so decomposed we were sticking to the floor. I'm really becoming irrational now, and I'm raving, "how bad does it suck, that someone could just die, and no one knows or gives a fuck?" "You just rot until the stench makes someone nauseous enough to think something is not right." "Then you're called to witness this disgust over and over and over." This night was really kicking my ass. I was still bitching as Matt left the station, but the icing on the cake was still yet to come.

I was working with a really nice lady. Her name was Dottie and we had worked well together before. She was very together and very low-key. As we were leaving the station, she could clearly sense my distress. She asked me to take is easy this morning and we would try not to work too hard. So we offer to back up BLS units all morning, on bullshit jobs, and this keeps us out of the real mix for awhile. At about one o'clock I'm looking to go out of service, when Central decides I haven't suffered enough yet. We get over to Harriet Tubman houses over on One–Four–Two for a trauma. A woman had gone out to cop some dope. In the fifth floor apartment, she left a one-year-old and a two-year-old being watched by a five-year-old girl. Well, whatever happened inside while the mother was gone will never be known, but the five-year-old girl wound up falling out of the window, five floors, onto the concrete side-walk below. So this girl was dead. Her head was completely cracked open and I could see tears in Dottie's eyes as we knelt over the broken child. Ten seconds seemed like eternity, as I listened to the sing song rhythmic tune of an ice cream truck coming up the block and getting stuck behind our ambulance. By now our concerned mother was run-ning back up the block yelling, "what happened?" "What happened?" She became hysterical as she saw what happened. There was nothing I could do. I had no miracles; I had nothing good to say. We transported the kid over to Harlem, and if I live to be nine hundred I can't ever forget this job.

When I left the station, for the first time I truly felt like I didn't give a shit about this job anymore. From now on, I was going to do the whole fucking endless process, for the paycheck, which wasn't exactly a great motivator.

CHAPTER 24

We had just gotten a new vehicle. 16–Victor was gaining a lot of respect and I had to practically get dirty knees for a brand new bus. It had less than five hundred miles on it. That night I came to work and found out Jason and I would be on the biggest piece of shit in service. The crew on tour three had been idling the rig outside the Harlem emergency room, when some crackhead walked up to this woman medic who was working on the unit that afternoon. He told her he had a gun, and to get out of the way. Well he didn't have a gun, but she gave him the unit. Anyway, this asshole got down the block and around the corner of a Hundred and Thirty-fifth Street, then totaled the ambulance between two parked cars. Then he drove up on the sidewalk and ran into the side of a building. So we had a new rig for a whole week, but now we were sentenced to ride a nag of a bus, while our stallion was in for long-term repairs. Now, I know she did the right thing by giving up the vehicle to this maniac, but that didn't stop me from bitching. I'm telling Jason, "what the fuck do you mean, he didn't even have a gun?" These are the streets of Harlem. So he's amused and he's eggin' me on as I continued, "if I gave up my shit every time someone said gimme it, I'd be fucking standing here naked."

So eventually I calmed down and we restocked our version of Chitty, Chitty, bang, bang. We got a huge lift in morale when I saw Lieutenant Lardass standing by the rear of the rig talking with Brendan. She was breaking his balls about something meaningless and I tell Jason, "watch this." I pump the gas pedal good, and make like the rig is having a little trouble turning over, then I cranked the ignition and floored the gas pedal. The ambulance roared to life, and belched out a tremendous black soot cloud, that completely engulfed the two of them. I pissed Brendan, and her off good and I told Jason, "guess who's getting mandated in the morning?" Well anyway, after the Lieutenant got done ripping my ass, I had Jason laughing so hard he was literally crying. I knew it was gonna be a fun night and I needed one. Then we got the fuck out of there before Brendan could stop gagging and come rip us too. We headed around the block and onto the triangle till Central decided to abuse us.

So I'm watching the clear sky and I'm thinking what fucked up thing can happen tonight that keeps the newspapers in business? Suddenly our pimp summons his favorite Harlem whore. "6–Victor." "Victor go" I answered. "One–Four–Seven and Convent for the unconscious, 3–Charlie on the back." I hear Derek tell Central he's responding, then I announce we're sixty-three. It takes longer to get up the five flights than it does for us to get there. The staircase is very narrow and winding. At least a dozen stairs are nothing more than wood slats over cracked, and deteriorated cement. Some have holes; your whole leg could fall through. Others are completely gone. When we get up into and old abused tenement lot we're met by an eighteen year old kid who's telling us he just got home from work, and his father is unresponsive. So he leads us to the back of the flat, and on the bed is this guy, close to four hundred pounds. He's conscious but incoherent. He's lying there completely naked and he's covered in sticky tarry, foul smelling shit. Which is only slightly more offensive than the actual garbage stink in the loft. So I get a look at this guy, and by this time we can hear Derek and Ziffy doing the mountain goat routine, to get to the loft. The son leaves to let the other crew in and I look over at Jason who's staring in disbelief at our patient. I ask him, "have you ever seen anything like this before?" He muttered, "no, but it looks like he's having a fucking baby". Well this guy had a long vast history of IV drug abuse. His whole body was edema filled. I don't know if he was in renal failure, liver failure, heart failure or all three. But his scrotum was as big as a soccer ball.

First, we had to figure out what was wrong with him. Then, we needed to figure how the fuck we were going to get him out of this rat hole. The stairs were way too narrow, and unsafe to carry him down. We called for a patrol supervisor, and Jimmy showed up. He advised us to call for a ladder company, so this guy could be cherry-pickered out the window. The firemen were gonna love us for this, but what the hell, an order is an order. Besides, these guys were getting paid more than us anyway. So we're thinking this guy's really fucked up, but his most pressing problem is kidney failure. He's got no IV access. This motherfucker used all his veins, including the junkie veins under the forearms, the veins in his feet and in his neck. He was gonna need a cut down central line in the emergency room and the son told us this is what happened the last time. Then Ziffy asked me, "does that mean this guy has been like this before?" Well anyway, Jason gives him a shot of narcan, and a shot of glucagon IM, cause he is AMS. But, we can't even get a flash for the line anywhere. I'm looking up top for anything I can hit, and Derek kiddingly says, "he's got a vein over here in his eyeball that I don't think he used up yet." It takes the firemen about thirty minutes, to get this guy out the window, and down to the street for us. When we get him on board our garbage skow, I intubated him with little resistance. Then we took him over to Columbia. After the job, the four of us are having coffee, and none of us could come up with a job like that in our past.

I told Ziffy that I had the vibe before we even left the station. He responded to me that Dano and Cato where in the house tonight. He was laughing as he left, and he told me, "we'll back the ninja medics all night." This made me feel good cause we we're getting big time respect from all the BLS units that backed us, and my hard work was really paying off inside me. So we're waiting for our next assignment. We'd already made all the big balls jokes you could think of, and it was time to get serious.

We hear PD get dispatched to One–Three–Five and Broadway (you guessed it, 3333) for a stabbing. We know the location, and we know it'll be real. It's just a matter of how bad. Jason doesn't need to be asked by me, he just starts heading over there, as I start to check my pouch for large bore IV's, and occlusive dressings. So we hear the PD unit start screaming over the air that, "we need EMS forthwith." By this time, we had already been dispatched along with 16–David. Our captain was on the patrol that night and being he was in the area he responded too. The captain was on the scene first and we pulled up from the south end of Broadway, as Jimmy and Tony sped down from the north side. I got out of the rig with my partner. We saw the captain standing over this twenty-year-old kid, who was on the ground in a huge puddle of blood that was spurting out his throat. The captain was pale. It was like he was turned to stone and couldn't move as his jaw hung down to his knees, and his thumb was jammed up his ass. The kid had tried to rob a chicken joint on the corner of One–Three–Five. The guy behind the counter stabbed him in the throat with a ten-inch carving knife, completely tearing it open. Anyway, Jason and I throw this guy on a board. Jimmy jumps to the front of our rig to drive and Tony is giving a traumatic arrest notification before we're even moving. We leave the BLS rig on the scene, with our fearless leader (who by the way passed the seventy-five question multiple choice test, qualifying him to wear the bars.). We took a straight hard ninety-second run down to St. Luke's. Tony did CPR, while Jason hit two fourteens on the fly. I did the tube, then tried to seal the wound. His throat was cut so bad; you could see the tube through the hole in his trachea. I knew this kid had no chance, but we worked like hell anyway. Ultimately, the grim reaper won another battle.

Our captain met us back at the station, as we were mopping out the rig, and doing restock. He told us we did a good job, but what else could he say. He would never bother me again after that job, as we both knew the truth. I had proved to him at money time, that Jason and I had game. While he had proved he was nothing more than a paper-pushing bureaucrat, who didn't belong on the street doing patient care. We went and got some dry hamburgers over on One–Two–Five then headed to the triangle. While I was eating, I was thinking about how electric these jobs used to make me, and how now all I wanted was for my tours to be over, before they even start. I was having trouble comprehending how so much could happen so fast, and how radically my feelings were changing. We laid low the rest of the night, staying busy on the BLS circuit. When the sun rose, I knew my pass days would soon arrive, but I would be back in a couple to start the whole fuckin' endless process again.

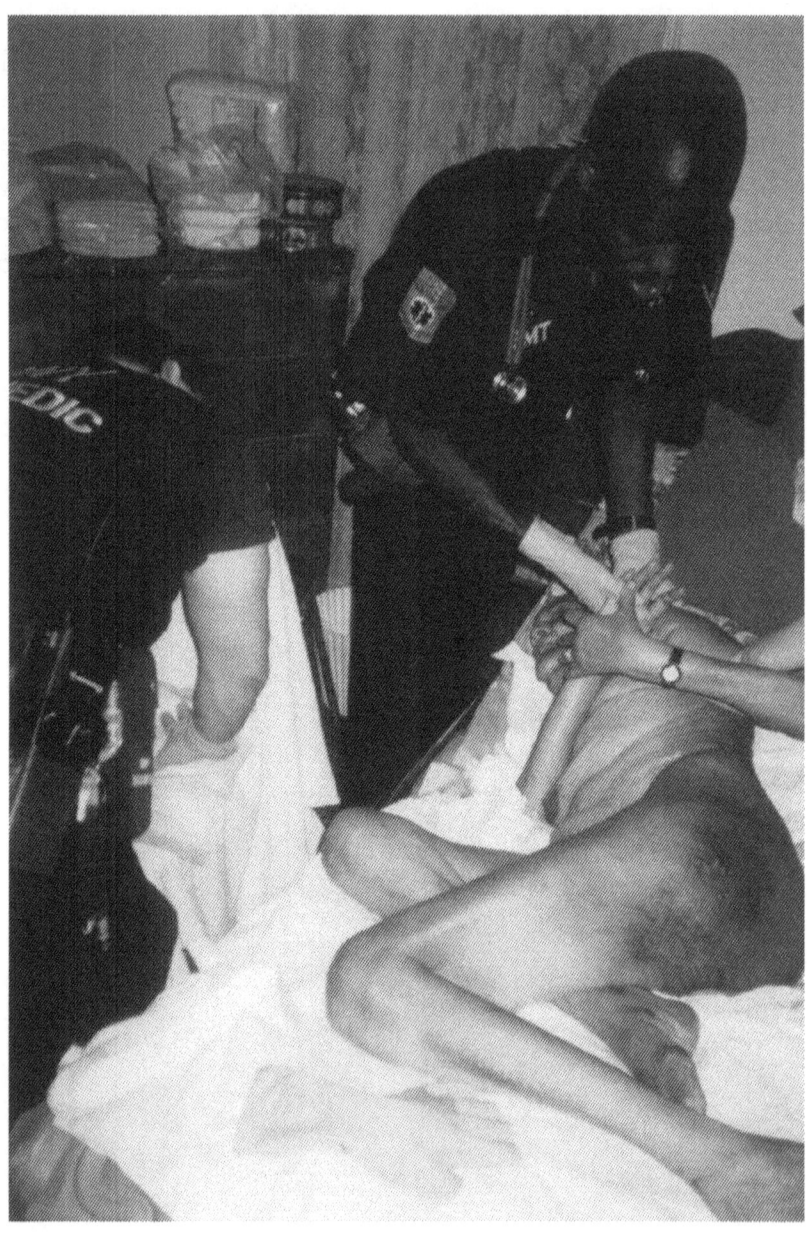

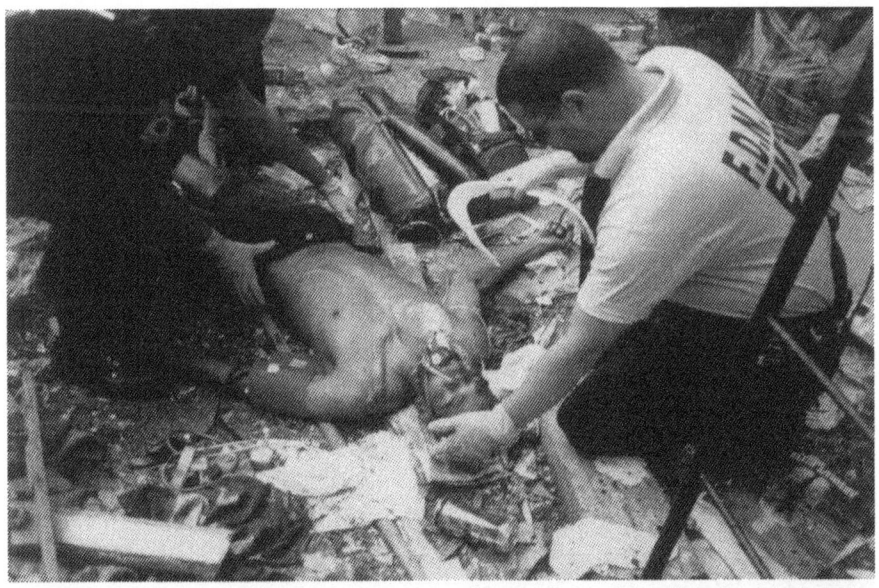

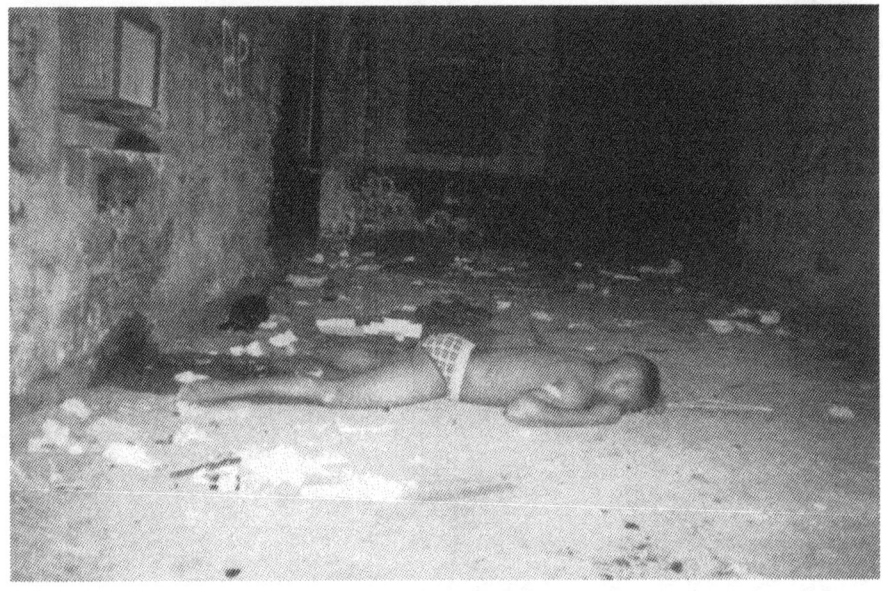

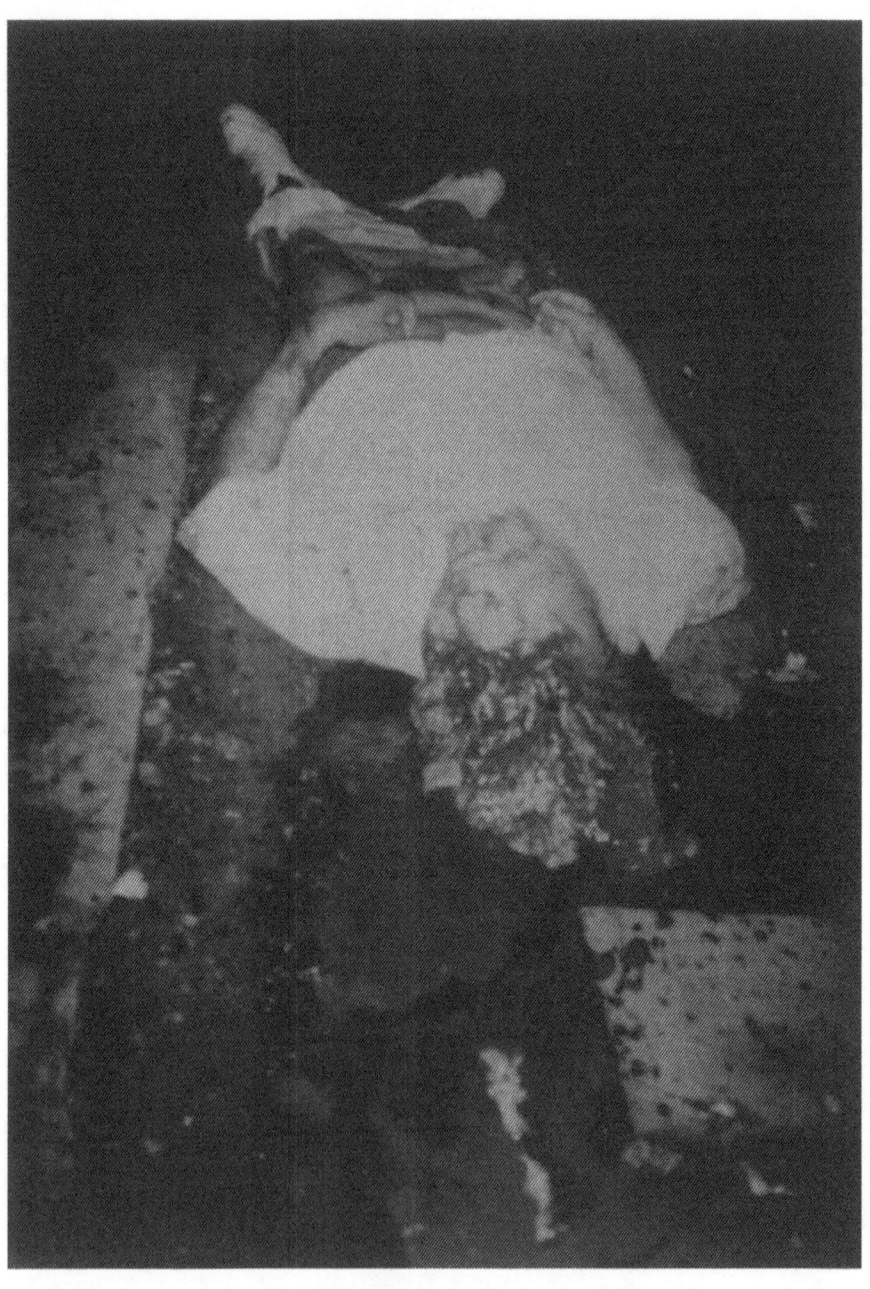

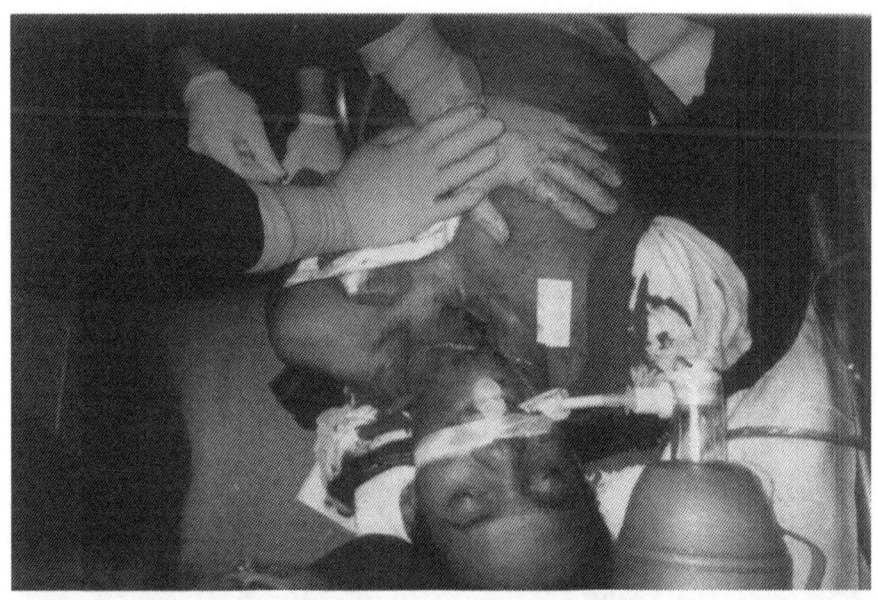

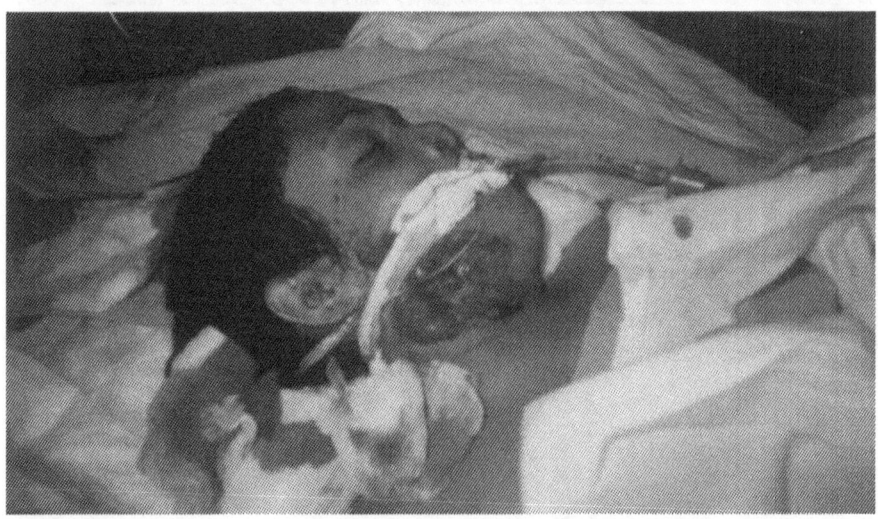

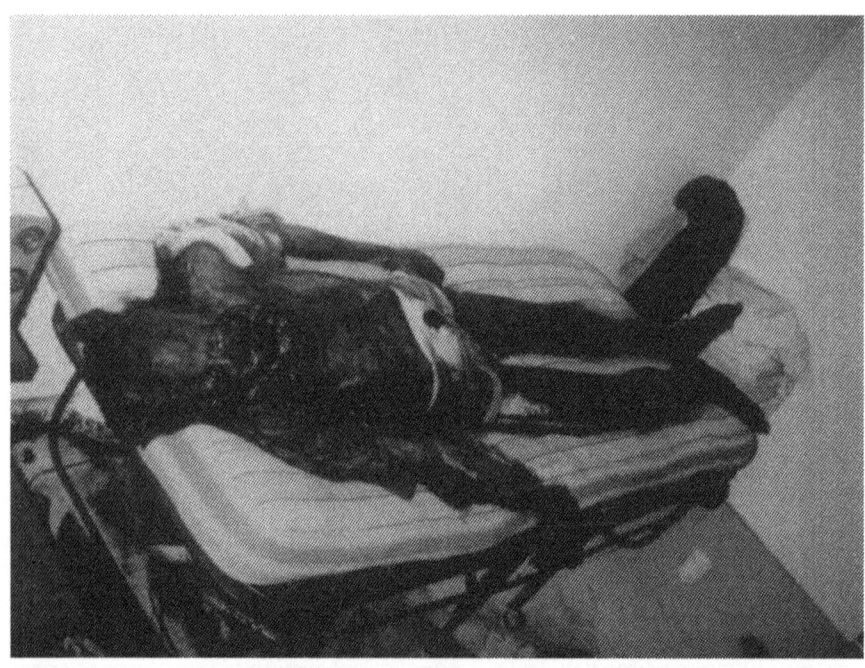

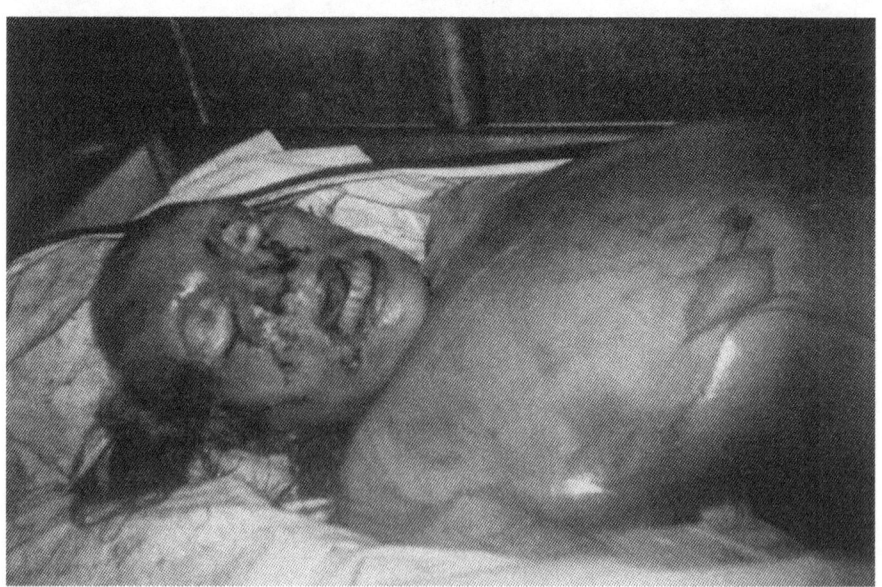

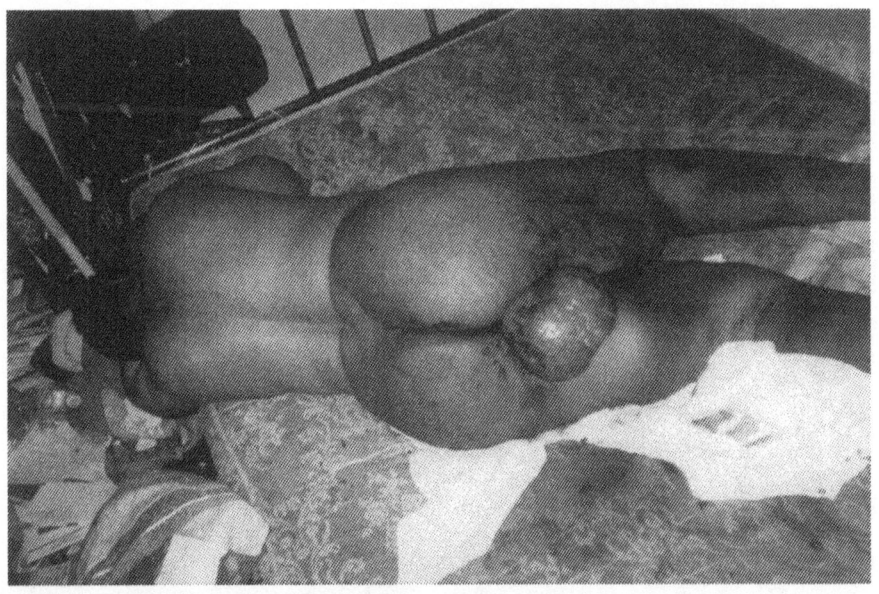

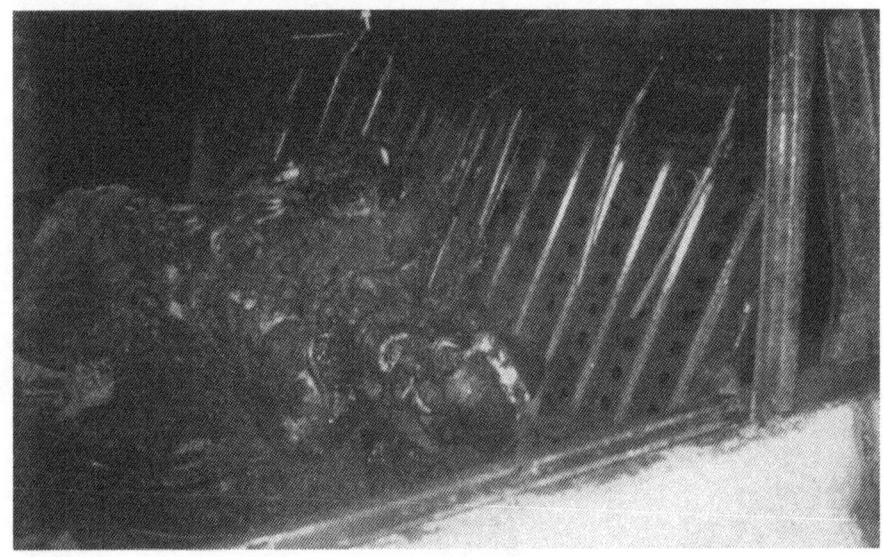

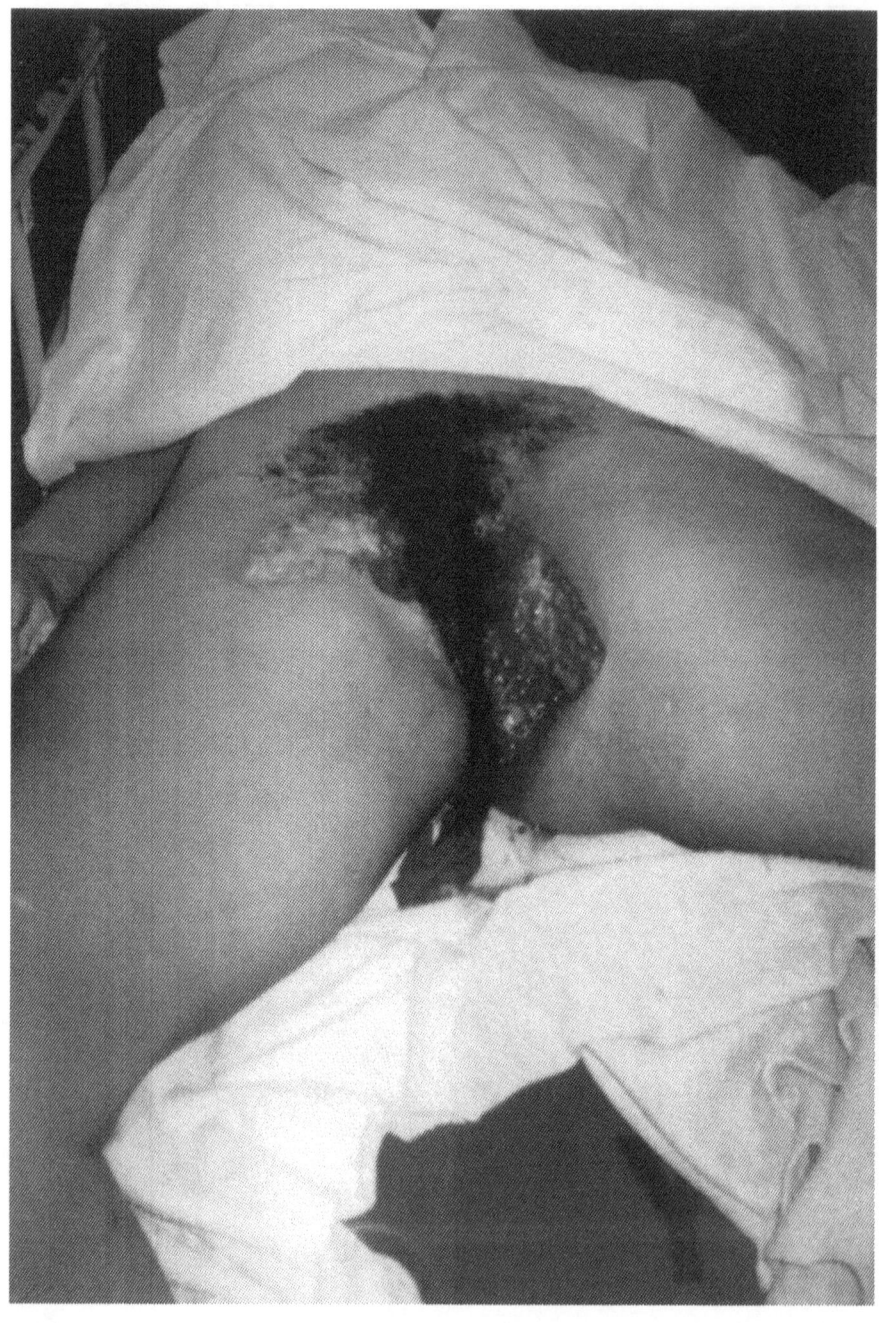

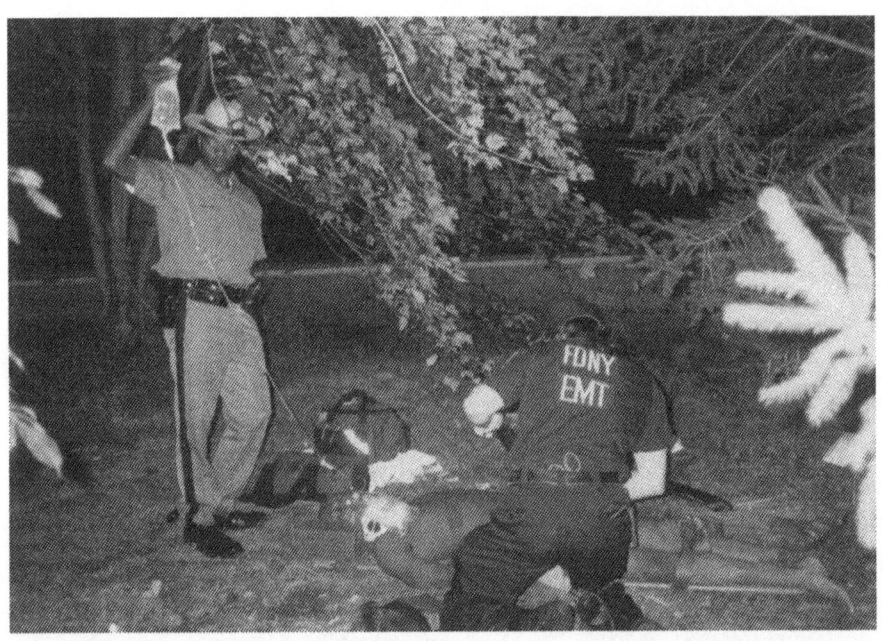

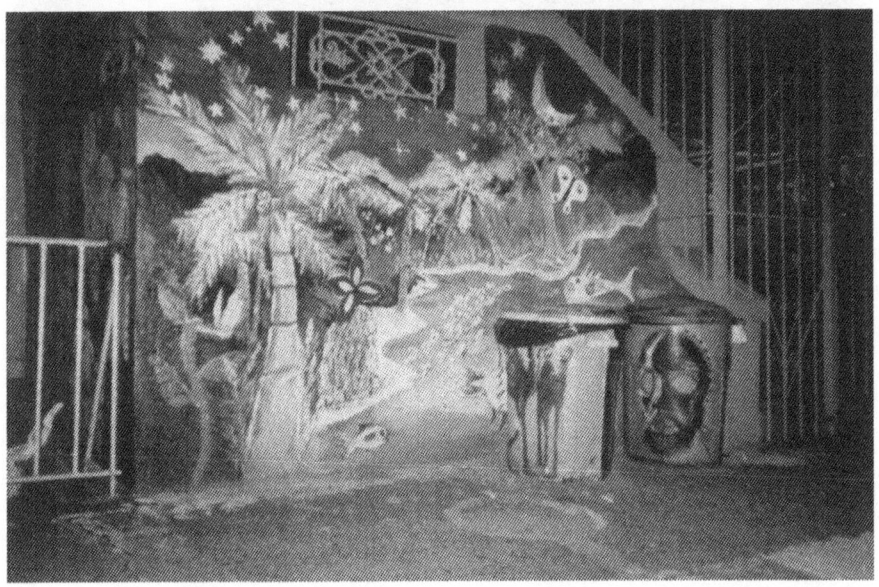

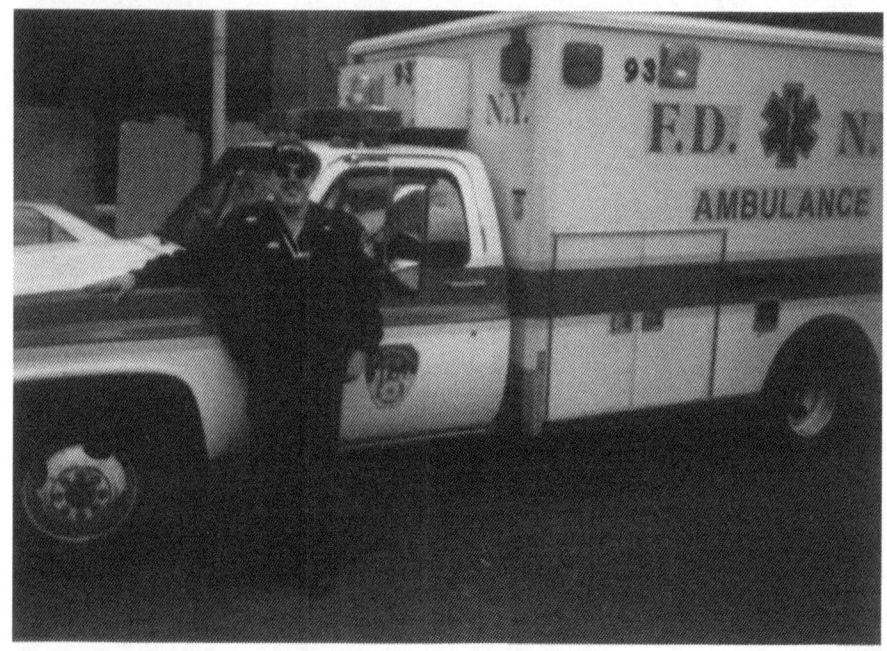

Pilot of the Starship Victor.

CHAPTER 25

I had a nice couple of nights off. For the most part, I just vegged out on the farthest piece of my property, under the trees and birdhouses. My neighbor came over, and we split a six-pack. She told me her and her husband had named this area the zone, and they knew when I was smoking in the zone that I had a bad night. The zone was a cool place. I built a crescent stone wall planter to seal off the corner of the fence. I planted all kinds of shrubs and vines, along with roses layered on and around the fences. I put two hundred and fifty bulbs in my planter and by now it was an explosion of assorted depths and colors. There were a few pine trees that I put in, a baby red oak and a red maple. Well anyway, I confirmed that things were pretty crazy on my job and that the zone was a good release. I'm pretty happy when I'm back here. Whether I'm working or recovering, the time off goes quickly. Then reality sets back in.

I get back to the grind and I'm gonna work with Matt. Jason has pass days and Rich has vacation time. So we ride on Matt's unit. It's a slower area and his rig is nice. Considering Victor would run in central Harlem and we would be on the old vehicle, the choice was easy. Well we get into service and head all the way up to our area, on One–Eight–Five and Broadway. But guess what? There's no Victor unit tonight. So we're parked about thirty seconds before Central sends us back down to One–Three–Two and Park for a difficulty breathing. We arrive on the scene, to find a thirty-eight-year-old woman, who tells is she has a history of SVT. We do her vitals, and sure enough her heart rate is over two hundred, and her blood pressure is 180/114. So we set up an IV, and got the adenosine ready. The first six-milligram bolus had no effect. I loaded up a twelve-milligram bolus, and Matt did the push. Our patient went flat-line for about five seconds, and slumped forward in the chair. Suddenly her eyes opened up, and she sat upright. She began to catch her breath, as the monitor showed a steady sinus rhythm at ninety-two. We took her over to North General where she was observed for a few hours, and then sent home without any complications.

When we were restocking the drug bag, I said to Matt, "I love to use adenosine, but it still freaks me out when they go under like that." We got back in service and we continued to discuss the virtues of a drug that stops your heart completely, as if it was a car doing one- twenty hitting a wall. Then, reboots it perfectly, as if nothing had happened at all. As our conversation ended, Matt asked me, if I liked adenosine as much as narcan? "Narcan was clearly my favorite", I said, being that it not only woke up near dead people, but it woke them up good enough to walk. So we head back up to Washington Heights, all the way up Broadway. We heard Junior and Richie B. get a job for an unknown condition up near us. We figured we'd back them up on it. This'll make us look good with them, and we won't get pulled back down another eighty blocks to Victor's area. So we get to the building, and as we pull up, I see Richie out on the second floor fire escape. He tells us he can see a guy on the floor of the living room having a seizure. The patient was alone in the apartment, and a neighbor said she heard strange noises through the wall which was actually her neighbor seizing uncontrollably. When no one answered the phone or the door, and the noises continued, she called 911. When Richie and Junior arrived, Richie went out on the fire escape through the neighbor's apartment window and was in the process of getting into the patient's living room through the window as we pulled up. We get up the stairs and Richie opens the door for us.

We find a sixty-three-year-old man flopping around on the rug, like a mackerel in the sand. We send Junior to find the meds in the bathroom then get the scoop stretcher. Matt goes to the phone to talk to medical control while me and Richie work on the patient. He steadies a swinging arm for me, and we drop a line in his hand. I push dextrose, narcan and thiamin to no avail. Matt comes back from his consultation with medical control and as ordered we push valium to end the seizure. Our patient is unresponsive at this time, so I intubated him. We get him packaged on the scoop, and carry him down to the rig. The four of us place the scoop onto the stretcher, and put the patient in the rig. I'm in the back with Matt, and I give Richie the keys to our bus. Low and behold it won't start. So this is great, we got this knocked out, intubated patient on board a dead bus. So we take the stretcher and the patient out, and wheel him over to Junior's rig, We put their empty stretcher on our broken vehicle, then put the patient on their bus. Richie gets his unit running, and Junior comes in the back with me and Matt. We leave the scene, and notify a patrol supervisor of our situation. As we're rolling towards CPMC, I'm asking Matt to "please explain to me how his brand new vehicle is dead already?" I didn't expect an answer and I didn't get one. We arrived at CPMC without further incident then got a ride back up to our vehicle to wait for roadside repair to come in from Queens, and get us rolling again.

We were out of service for about an hour for repairs then we still needed to restock our narcotics, and equipment. So it was a nice little vacation. We had done a good job, and I knew Richie appreciated us backing him without even being assigned to the job initially. We leave the station and jump on the drive to head back uptown. As we started heading up, we see a make shift shanty, blazing on the side of the highway, lighting up the river. So we pull over to the side of the road and ask Central to dispatch an engine to the scene. This hut was nothing but dry scrap wood, which had been baking all summer in the sun. By the time we saw it, it was already fully involved. When it was extinguished, we found a roasted body in a wheel chair. All that was left was a blackened skeleton completely roasted from the soles of his feet to the point of his head. This job kept us out of service for another hour as the night was now on cruise control heading to morning.

After BLS had removed the crispy critter from the side of the highway, we were hoping to get up to the Cloisters, and nod out for a bit. If the EMS god was smiling today, maybe we wouldn't get another job. Maybe we would get in for the change on time. Maybe we wouldn't get mandated and maybe there wouldn't be traffic going home. Then again maybe I would hit the lotto and I wouldn't have to come back to these fucked up situations. So as we attempted to head uptown, Matt is getting all philosophical on me, and we're trying to figure out why the fuck we do this job anyway. I said that I believed in a way this was a destiny, almost like the Quantum Leap guy. You know, fix what was once wrong; try to positively affect someone's future, and all that happy nonsense. As we pulled off the drive at One–Seven–Eight, he looked across at me and said, "oh you mean we're just destined to be God's janitors." For once, I didn't answer him I just looked out the window across the river and thought about if my buddies in the Bronx where having a wonderful time too.

So the sun rises, as we get an assignment down in the Port Authority bus terminal. "13–Charlie, 13–X-ray, One–Seven–Nine and Broadway for the unconscious," Central commands. Ziffy and Derek are backing us on this one, and they arrive on the scene before us. As we pull up, Derek gets on the air to ask for an ETA, and tells us he's got an OD in the women's bathroom deep in the terminal. Anyway, PD leads us through, up a flight of stairs and another five hundred feet or so further in.

When we get in, we got this tremendous woman, well over three hundred pounds, zonked out on the toilet, with the needle still in her arm Her pants and underwear are down to her ankles, revealing a nightmare of roll upon roll of blubbery belly hanging over vericosed thunder thighs. I was quick to think to flush the toilet before we removed her off it. I had trouble reaching around her to get to the lever. Well the cops are wondering, how the fuck we're gonna get her out of there. And I ask

Derek, "should request a forklift?" The cops think I'm serious and are asking me, "how are you gonna get a forklift up the stairs and in here?" "I'm not," I laughed, watch this. I asked Matt, "hey buddy what's your favorite drug narcan or adenosine?" I took three bristo jets from the bag, as I removed the syringe from our patient's arm I hot shotted two milligrams into the vein she had already polluted. Then I took the other two bristos and gave them IM one in a flabby, dangling tricep. Then just for the hell of it, one in the side of her ass. It took about four minutes, but little by little she came around, and started to talk to us. She was just another Jersey jerkoff, who came over to cop in the middle of the night, and couldn't get back in time to be Fort Lee's problem. Anyway, she gets up off the bowl and tries to start walking while her legs are still tangled in her clothes. So in order to avoid an earthquake and potential trauma to the building we help her get dressed. As she waddles to the vehicle, the cops are as grateful as we are for narcan, and one of them is asking Derek what it was we gave her. I said, "miracle N," the same time Derek said, "pharmaceutical forklift." Even Matt, the eternal stoic, cracked a smile as we headed out of the building.

We dropped off queen mobey at CPMC and got in for the change on time. I didn't get mandated, and I cruised home with no problem. I smoked some hydro's, while my radio pumped out Live at Leeds. Maybe I should buy a lottery ticket, I said to myself as the instrumental of My Generation kicked in. I cruised the open road without another vehicle in sight and for a while, I forgot about the whole fucking endless process.

Chapter 26

When I came into work with Jason tonight, we were pleasantly surprised to find out that our unit had been repaired, and was back in service and already on the road. The tour three guys were on a late job, and this was good for us, cause it sounded like we would need to do some extensive restock when they got back. We wouldn't be in service until after one o'clock. Which I figured took twelve and a half percent of my tour right off the top. So Mark and Steve had done a double shooting over by colonial park houses. From what Mark described it was pretty messy and gang related. He warned me that we would probably be scraping up the repercussions before sunrise. I mentioned are you gonna help me scrape the initial percussions out of the rig. So as he was about to leave I asked, "come on, how many times are you gonna get time and a half to hose out brain matter?" "Too many," be responded as be headed wearily towards the parking lot. So after we clean the rig, Jason and I offer Steve a ride to the train station. He was still pretty upset over his late job and he told us, "they were both just kids." We had already heard they both died, so neither of us talked too much. We let Steve get it out, and told him to get home safe, after dropping him off.

Central was calling us for an assignment. We get sent over to One–Four–Seven and Amsterdam for a traumatic arrest. We got Richie and Junior backing us, and the KDT is showing that, PD is requesting at a crime scene to pronounce. So Jason looks at me with it's gonna be one of those nights stares, as we let Central know we're responding. We arrive on the scene the same time as BLS. As we step into the vertical urinal to ascend up to the sixth floor, we're talking about Steve's earlier job and I'm saying I don't think its close enough to the projects to be related. Anyway, we step out of the elevator and theirs already like ten cops and six detectives there, and before we even get in, Richie is saying, "this is gonna be fucked up." Well this scene was completely unrelated to the previous shooting, but it was something right out of Scarface. We had a Dominican male corpse about thirty-five who was tortured, then had his head lopped off with a chainsaw. Before he was decapitated, he had his fingers cut off with a garden pruner, then he was sliced with a razor about a hundred and fifty times, while someone flicked gasoline into the open wounds. I guess when they couldn't possibly inflict any more pain on this guy, they cut his head off. Which we were told, was found out on the sidewalk in front of the building with its mouth duct taped shut, about a half-hour ago. Anyway, this was just another lesson in, never fuck the Dominicans for drug money, or whatever else this guy could have done. So by now I've learned how to block this shit out but Junior isn't so lucky yet. We leave to finish our paperwork downstairs. Richie knows his partner is pretty shook and the three of us talked with him for about twenty minutes, before me and Jason left, and Richie went back to the station with his partner for awhile.

We're back in service and we decide we should hang on the Washington Heights, Harlem border, around One–Four–Five and Edgecombe or thereabouts. This is the place to be, cause the shit is hitting the fan around here all night, and the trauma hawks are out. We can be in the projects or in the Heights in under a minute from this location and our instincts are right, as Central sends us to One–Four–Six and Bradhurst for a shooting. We get there in under thirty seconds as we had just about picked the spot. We were right on the other side of the park by the public pool and we were so close I was surprised we didn't hear the shots. Anyway, it's a street job—a payback from before. This kid about sixteen is shot four times close range in the chest. He has multiple exit wounds, but he's alive and he's still talking. We get him on the rig and he's clutching my arm tightly repeating, "don't let me, die...don't let me die" as Jason starts to bang a couple of fourteens in him.

Richie and Junior had backed us up from the station. I heard on my portable radio, "16–David, show me on the scene of 16–Victor's job" as I looked out the back of my rig and saw Richie screeching to a halt next to our vehicle. He jumped in the back and I gave him our keys. He drove over to Harlem Hospital as me and Jason worked on the fly, and the notification was given. I told myself this one is not fucking dying on me. I was determined not to let him arrest. But in actuality this was far beyond my control. I kept the kid talking and set up a tube, just in case. Jason pumped up the blood pressure cuff around the bag of saline, and he infused as much fluid as possible. I let him know that I had no lung sound on the right side as we were pulling around on One–Three–Six and were about twenty seconds from the emergency room. We got this kid inside and I watched the doctor do a chest tube while the kid was still awake. They took about two pints of blood out of his lungs and I was amazed at how this kid was still alive let alone conscious and screaming. He was even able to give a brief description of his assailant to the detectives.

A few months later, we were called to testify on the grand jury as witnesses for the prosecution. Our patient had survived, and I remember feeling like this was the job where I found myself that in spite of all the concentrated, repetitive misery. This is where I belong. This is what I was supposed to be doing and that the good of having been busted six years ago was showing itself now. I was proud to be a Harlem medic, and I was proud that 6–Victor was my unit. As much as I hated my job, I felt needed and productive and in a backward sort of way I also loved my job. I always wondered though how long I could teeter on the border of burnout insanity. As this really was an endless fucking process.

CHAPTER 27

So some time has passed and things are going very well for me. I stay busy with my kids, and the job is a constant, who-knows-what's-next challenge. I'm frequently up in the dead of night wondering what the fuck my purpose is. I mean billions and billions of lost souls throughout time, struggling just for shelter or a meal, destroyed families, and lives being held together with nothing more than spit and glue. So even though I recognize that things are going good, it's still a struggle just to stay happy. I can barely take care of myself, but somehow I'm supposed to come up with medical miracles and psychological first aid for every lost person this machine of a city can spit up at me. I want to be religious and I believe that good is more powerful than evil, it's just that the bad things are so much more noticeable and my faith is shaky at best.

So Jason sees that I'm down, he's a really good guy, but even with a crane he's not going to be able to lift my spirits tonight. We talk about my new house and healthy kids, everything is in place for me to be happy. So how come I'm borderline suicidal at times? I don't know, but I just keep fighting like everyone else. We've been on the rig a few minutes and we get dispatched over to One–Two–Seven and Powell for an abdominal pain. These are the types of jobs that set me off. I can't believe people are actually allowed to call an ambulance for a bellyache. So I sarcastically call back to Central, that we're sixty-three, responding to the constipation, and I tell my dispatcher that I didn't restock the ex-lax tonight. I'm told to keep my comments off the air and respond to the job. So as we're about five blocks away, Central calls us for a higher priority, they try to turn us around and bring the unit up to One–Six–O and Riverside for a difficulty breathing, but I state that I'm already on the scene of my bellyache. "Fuck `em," I tell Jason. "They should think of these things before we get sent for bullshit." Anyway, there's no accountability. Central can send us anywhere they want. We can get a kid with a splinter, and if there's a cardiac arrest two minutes later with no medics available, se la vie.

So we climb up the stairs to a dirty, second floor apartment. We get a typically ignorant thirty-six year old woman, who hasn't taken a shit in three days. So now the whole fucking world has to stop for her. I wish they had enemas in protocol. Then, I wouldn't have felt so bad, when I heard Ziffy over the air, telling Central they were running over to CPMC, with a pulmonary edema patient. The same patient that there were no medics available for, because so many fucking idiots took us all out of service with hemorrhoids, bellyaches, and hangovers. Anyway, by now I wasn't exactly the most compassionate guy in the world. I strapped our patient on the bench, right over the wheel well, I asked Jason if I could drive, because I didn't feel like even talking to this person. So he gives me the keys and I decide I'll hit every fucking pothole I can find, and if I miss any I'll back up over them. As I make turns, I'm sure to run over the curbs, just to make sure our patient was going to remember the ride. When we get to Harlem Hospital, I'm so pissed off I don't even get out of the vehicle. I let Jason walk our girl in, and I chain-smoked four cigarettes while he took care of the paper work.

So the night goes on while the system keeps churning out bullshit for us. At about four-thirty in the morning, I thought I was awake but I must've been in that twilight sleep, we seemed to live on. The radio startled me as we were getting sent down to One–Fourteen and Douglas for another abdominal pain. The KDT told us we had a thirteen-year-old girl and I was so annoyed I couldn't even see straight. This is what I meant when I said there was so much bullshit you could actually get beaten down by it, and be caught off guard. I'm raving, "go to the clinic in the morning or take a fucking cab," as we cruise down Eighth Avenue.

We get to the scene and this guy about twenty-five lets us into the apartment. He tells us he doesn't know what's the matter, but something is suspicious. Anyway, it turns out this girl is mad pregnant. Normal people will find this hard to believe, but no one in the house knew she was pregnant, but guess what, the secret was out now. She was such a little girl; she really looked only twelve or thirteen, except for her small bowling ball of a belly. She didn't tell anyone of her problem, and it was as if Guy Lombardo was doing the countdown when we made patient contact. I felt nauseous as I knew we were gonna deliver this baby's, baby. While the whole time, the guy has got this stupid smile like everything is all right and this is a good thing. The mother or aunt or whoever the fuck she was, is actually yelling at the little girl, "how could you do this to me," as the baby is being delivered.

After this job I had a lot of paperwork to complete. Lieutenant Lardass was on the desk tonight and when we went back to the station, I was telling her I didn't feel well. She was actually pretty human tonight and she was asking me if I thought I could finish the tour. I said that I would try, but at that moment I couldn't contain my nausea anymore. I was about to leave the office when I projectile vomited all over the place. I got to the garbage can as the last of my fried rice came up. There's no janitor on the overnights, so I had to clean my own mess. I got sent home sick a couple of hours early and I didn't even take my uniform home. I just got changed then slam-dunked my shirt and pants into a garbage can. It was still dark out, as I headed over the George Washington Bridge, and up the Palisades. My decision was made. I had to get the fuck out of this place soon or I really was going to go postal.

I made arrangements with Jason to do a double later in the week, we rigged it so we would do sixteen hours, then get an extra pass day. Which was my version of pay now, sleep later. We came in at four o'clock to pilot Victor 'till morning. I knew it was gonna be a long night, so I took my time getting in service. It was a little before five when we got assigned to a drowning on Ward's Island. I hated this place. I called it the island of bad feet. This was nothing more than a giant homeless shelter; an island in the middle of the East River, with row upon row of cubicles and beds. The place always smelt like fungus, and here is where our liberal and caring city attempted to hide it's less fortunate and those without a place to go. Anyway, this shelter is notorious for bullshit jobs, and overdoses. I frequently was amazed at how someone could have no money, no place to go, and no food, but they were able to OD on heroin or something. Anyway, this time we never got into the building. As we pulled up to the scene with PD, we were led down to the water's edge, on the rocks that formed the seawall around the island. We found a bloated male corpse bobbing in the water, washed up on the rocks. Jason looked down and said to me, "he ain't doing the backstroke is he?" as we climbed down and got a closer look. I notified Central that we had a DOA and would need harbor patrol for a removal, as I finish speaking into the radio. I told the cops he had been in the drink for about two weeks. He had seaweed stuck in his eye, and I observed that the guy was wearing a New York Knicks sweatshirt, and that the watch on his wrist was still working. I had Jason hysterical as I did my impersonation of the Timex man, standing on a rock over our floater, "yes folks, there you have it, it takes a dipping and keeps on ticking." We did the paperwork, snapped a couple of photos for the family album, then moved on as harbor did the cleanup.

So we head across town over to One–Ten. I guess the smell of all that fresh saltwater air put me in the mood for my lox and cream cheese, on an onion bagel. We weren't too busy the rest of the evening, and we coasted toward midnight with an assortment of uneventful nonsense, and unworthy transports. We rolled the unit over at midnight, as our designation changed from 16–Victor–3 to 16–Victor–1. It had been an annoying but easy first half, and I was getting happy now, cause I knew I couldn't get mandated today, and all I had to do was survive the next eight hours. Then I would have four nights off. The way things had been going I would be doing a lot of gardening over the next couple of days.

So a little before one, we hear Rosa and Mary get a job for an OB complication, on One–Fourteen, up by St. Nick. They had been on the scene for a while, and I pretty much wasn't paying no mind to what the other units were doing. So I was kinda surprised when I heard Rosa screaming into the radio, that she had a newborn arrest and needed medics forthwith. Nobody needed to be dispatched to this, because she wasn't even done talking before we had banged a U-turn off the triangle on One–Three–Six and sped down St. Nicholas Avenue. I came up on the air and announced to Central that 6–Victor was less than a minute away, show us six-three, responding. The ladies had delivered a stillborn baby girl to a junkie. The mother was high when she went into labor, and it was another one of those jobs where, as the baby was popping out, someone decided this would be a good time to call 911.

So we're jettin' up the stairs, as the girls are coming down. Mary's got the oxygen bag, and Rosa has a blue baby girl cradled in her arms, while she's trying the ventilate, and get down to her rig. So we pick them off in the staircase, and Rosa is in a frenzy. They left the mother upstairs, and another BLS crew was dispatched for her. I'm saying to her, "calm down, we been here before, we're gonna get this done."

So we get into Victor's bus, and place the newborn on a short board. We left our unit running and it was toasty warm in back. Rosa did rapid CPR with the tips of two fingers, and Jason was setting up an intra osseous line, as I grabbed a 2.5 ET tube from the peds set. I opened up the baby's tiny mouth, and carefully slid the tube in a microdot of a trachea. The first part was done. The next thing was to stay focused, and not let my own adrenaline blow out her lungs, by over squeezing the bag I was now going to use, to give this baby the first breaths of her life. I sent the first breath down and immediately the main problem presented itself, as a load of amniotic fluid came up the tube, as a result of the positive pressure the oxygen provided. The girls hadn't suctioned the newborn adequately, and she aspirated with her first breath. I pulled the full tube back out, and I said to Jay, "I need a new tube, and .3 of narcan." He looked back at me, and said quickly, "I'm a little busy right now", as he screwed the IO into place.

I wasn't about to play games now. The rig was getting trashed, and the shit was really circling the bowel. So I looked over at him, then at he tube in my hand. I blew through it, clearing it of all fluid, not the most sterile of techniques, I'll admit, but effective. I placed it back through the tiny vocal chords and squeezed a breath in and the process repeated itself, as more fluid came up the tube. By now Jason had sent a tiny bolus of narcan through the baby's fibula. After I cleared the ET a second time, I placed it back into the small pink slot, between vocal chords, no larger than a daisy petal. By now, we were on the fly, up St. Nicholas to One–Three–Six, then down to Harlem. Mary had left the BLS rig on the scene, and was giving an arrest notification as we were rolling. I squeezed the bag a couple of times, and then revisualized the placement. I saw the vocal chords start to open and close around the baby's lifeline. In that split second, everything in the world seemed all right, as the child was starting to breathe on her own. I extubated the baby and continued to use the bag to provide oxygen. When we got to the ER, we had a pink, warm baby girl. Everyone in the ER was standing around the crash cart wearing their penitentiary faces. Well faces of doom soon turned to smiles, as it became clear this kid was gonna make it. Needless to say the rest of my night breezed. I was on one of the all time highs of my man-icness. When I got home for my long weekend, I did all my gardening out of pleasure and not frustration, and I remember thinking on that morning that the whole fucking endless process wasn't all bad.

CHAPTER 28

So it's been a pretty wild summer, forget about full moons and other nonsense. The crazies are out every night, all night. The grind has taken its toll and if I were to live to be 900, I wouldn't be able to forget this shit. So I'm working tonight with this guy from the Bronx, named Elvis. He's a tour three guy that I went through the academy with and we know each other very well. I was very flattered because he came to work over-time at Harlem with me. He knew tonight there would be a vacancy on my unit and we would be able to work together. So Elvis is a big bald, no nonsense Spanish guy. He's very street smart and a little grissomed from working in the South Bronx. He likes to work hard. So even though he's on overtime, I know we're not gonna skell, and I'm looking forward to showing him the sights of 16–Victor, along with its finest cuisine available in the middle of the night.

So I get us in service quickly and we head over to White Castle on One–Two–Five for some belly bombs, and French fries that tastes more like wood chips than potatoes. We get a call for a chest pain over on One–Two–Two and Manhattan Avenue. I immediately know who this is, but I'm playing dumb as I say to Elvis, "this could be a real MI." We better make some time as I stick our sack of burgers behind the seat and light up the rig.

When I pull us up to the scene there's Otis, standing on the corner holding his little overnight suitcase with one hand and the center of his chest with the other like he's pledging allegiance. So I tell Elvis, "go ahead you talk to him, see what's up." Well, Elvis introduces himself to our frequent flyer and asks Otis, "what's the problem tonight." So Otis looks across at me while brushing off Elvis, he's staring silently for about a second before he mutters, "god damn fucking rookies, why don't you go over there and ask your partner how I'm a sick man with a heart condition." "He knows, now take me to the damn hospital and don't be touching me either and don't ask me no more questions." I asked Otis to go easy on my rookie partner. I wink at Elvis as I finish, "you know how it is breaking in these kids." I gently helped him into the rig and let him sit on the stretcher. I didn't need to ask anything, as I had his name, address, birthday and even social security number committed to memory now. I even drew in a stable set of consistent vitals and Otis got what he needed; a quiet, uneventful taxi ride over to his second home, St Luke's.

So the nurse initials my paperwork and Otis goes over to the waiting area to watch TV for a few hours, as his chest pain now seems to have miraculously dissipated. As we left I said to Elvis, "I'll do him tomorrow with Jason, then Brendan or Matt the day after." Then we went back in service and headed up Amsterdam toward City College to finish eating. So we get parked for about two minutes. I had inhaled a couple more burgers as we heard PD get dispatched to an MVA over on One–Two–O and Riverside by Grant's Tomb. I flipped on the lights and started to head that way while I waited for the job to come over EMS. Richie and Junior got the assignment and I asked Central to put us on their back. We let them get on the scene first and as we pulled up, Richie and Elvis recognized each other from their years in the South Bronx. They quickly exchanged greetings as Elvis said to Richie, "just like the old days when you used to back me up on Two–O Victor." Richie nodded approval as we walked up on a ninja motorcycle under a taxicab. A six-teen-year-old kid wiped out going around the turn, apparently trying to beat the red light. He went head on into the cab, as the bike slid under the front end. Our Spanish Evil Knevil went up and over the cab, breaking the windshield and then continuing until he landed about twenty feet to the rear of the taxi.

The taxi driver was uninjured, but he was really pissed because his vehicle was out of service now, and to use his own words, this pen de jo was gonna cost him a nights pay. Well the kid is pretty fucked up. His most immediate problem is that the chin strap of his helmet had cut into his throat and he was fortunate that it didn't go too much deeper or he would have been a DOA for Junior and Richie to take down to the morgue. He was wearing knee hi shorts and a cut tee shirt, which offered no protection what so ever, leaving him with extensive body wide road rash. We immobilized him on a board with the collar, then taped a non-rebreather on him. So his vitals are stable and the main concern is basically bleeding control and infection precautions, but no matter what we did those scrapes were gonna ooze puss for about three weeks.

Richie did the right thing by us, and took the transport, while we helped out a little further, then took the eighty-seven with our thanks. When we went back in service, I mentioned to Elvis that I thought Richie was a stand up guy in spite of what some people had to say. Elvis responded that he knew him from numerous jobs and he was an excellent EMT and as sincere, true to his inner voice person, as we drove away. I finished by saying, I always examine the source of things, if certain people don't like you, it's probably a validation of self and a good thing. We still had a couple of burgers left, but by now they would be better suited to be used to repair missing bricks in a wall than as food. So I tossed them out the window for the pigeons as we cruised back up Riverside Drive. We stopped by CPMC and bullshitted with Tom and Brendan for a bit, while I grabbed a couple of coffees and a pack of smokes. We killed about a half-hour before our dispatcher caught up to us and sent us all the way back down to One–Two–Two and Lexington for a multi-trauma job.

We got to the scene and found a Spanish guy about twenty-one. He was completely fucked up and had the mark of the rat carved into him—a deep jagged slash from the tip of his ear, to the edge of his lips.

He was left lying in the gutter like a piece of disposable garbage and a few different witnesses said the guy had come running out of the subway with about seven or eight other guys chasing him. We were told that he was beaten brutally with sticks and bottles, and someone even picked up the trash can on the corner and was smashing him with that. So this guy can't talk to us being that his jaw was broken and kinda dangling, giving him a contorted caricature type face. The slash was clean through his cheek and you could see into his mouth from the outside. When the blood had stopped, spit still continued to foam out of the wound. So we get him on the board and in the bus. I ask Elvis if he wants to do the tube or the line and he takes the start kit for the IV. We should've had a back up on this job, but things were getting busy and we were hung out on our own.

So I bang an 8.0 in him and as I open his mouth it was as I suspected, completely unhinged with no resistance. Elvis banged a fourteen in him and saw that all his fingers had been broken in addition to the numerous other injuries. We figured one line was good for now, and that we were already on the scene long enough. I went to the front to drive as Elvis took control of the tube, and continued to hyperventilate our patient. I got us over to Harlem Hospital and after completing the paperwork spoke with the cops for a bit. Our patient had no ID, but apparently somebody must've known who he was, because obviously he had spoken to the wrong people.

It took us about twenty minutes to get restocked and cleaned up. I could see Elvis was tired but we still had a couple of hours to go. So I headed us up One–Two–Five past the Apollo Theater and then the Cotton Club. I drove the rig under the Henry Hudson over-pass and parked us right on the river. The EMS god must've really been smiling on us today because even though it was still pretty busy we never got another job. We both fell asleep by the water and the morning sun shining on my forehead woke me up at about seven. Elvis was over on the passenger side, snoring like a Kawasaki. I didn't have the heart to wake him up. So I just called Central and put us out of service overtime personnel. I sat another fifteen minutes then headed us back toward the station. Elvis woke up as the vehicle started moving over the cobblestones. I let him know that we were done for the night and that I fixed it, so that by the time we got back and finished putzing around, he would get paid overtime for the full eight hours. As we left, we made arrangements for me to come work overtime on his unit in the Bronx. I laughed as I said, I remember what happened the last time I was there, and he told me don't worry Cherise moved to Florida last year. As he started his car and we temporarily parted ways.

CHAPTER 29

The summer is winding down and thankfully, the kids will be back in school. The cooler temperatures are a welcome relief and I'm doing a double today, overnight with Matt, then I'm gonna work tour two with Jason. He and Sophie did a mutual earlier in the week so Jason could have Friday night off with his girl, but he had to give Sophie a weekend day in return. I was next up to get mandated so I figured I would just volunteer to work with my partner, rather than be at the mercy of Lieutenant Lardass, as to who I worked with or what unit I was on.

When I got to work, I was about a half-hour late. I hadn't counted on overnight construction on the bridge and this set me back. Matt had already gotten the unit ready to go in service. And as we signed out our narcs, he told me that Tom and Rich got banged for a stat epp on One–Four–One and Powell. This was the heart of my area and Tom hated picking up my jobs there. So we got into service quickly and I asked Matt if he minded picking up a job for them later. We drove up One–Four–Five towards the bank over on Amsterdam so I could use the ATM. I was broke and since I had been late, I didn't get a chance to stop before work. Well I let myself into the little hall area with five ATM's, using my card. I was heading toward the one in the middle when I looked up and decided I would just use the first one, down on the end.

These two skinny crackheads were pushed together tightly into the little booth type area, at the other end. Anyway, I was minding my own business as I put my card in the machine. I glanced over to my right and sure enough the guy had the girl bent over on the screen and was ramming her slowly from behind. I got my money and walked out. They paid me no mind whatsoever as they continued a steady grind. When I got back to the rig I had one of those I thought I've seen everything looks. Matt asked what was wrong and all I said was back up about twenty feet, and look through the window. These two weren't noticeable unless you were looking. But sure enough, Matt cracks a big smile and asks, "are they having sex in there?" I responded, "yeah, I think they are." Then he asked me if I needed to go somewhere else to get money. I gave him a sarcastic stare and asked, "you're kidding right?" "Come on lets go eat before dispatch decides to bend us over." So after munching out on some Popeye's spicy fried chicken, we get a call for a difficulty breathing up in Esplanade Gardens off One–Four–Six. As we go sixty-three, Ziffy and Derek jump on our back and meet us over by the building.

We head up to the twentieth floor and get into a clean well-kept apartment. So the four of us are led in together by a large woman in her fifties. She's telling us she's been having a hard time catching her breath all day and its steadily getting worse. So we're in there and this woman has got a really hot daughter, who Ziffy immediately notices and starts to get a history from, while Matt continues to speak with our patient. She was acting really weird and must have been very hypoxic, but we hadn't figured that out yet. So the patient walks backwards till she hits the wall hard with her back, then continues to do this rhythmically about one smack every second. I ask her why she's doing this and she responds that it makes her feel better and her daughter confirms to Zif that her mother had been doing this all day and insinuated that this wasn't normal. So this woman is whacking herself against the walls hard. All the pictures are crooked and I'm noticing the rest of the apartment is really neat. So we're thinking this woman has gone EDP or something and no one's really taking her too serious yet. I ask her to please have a seat and I give her some oxygen as I ask if I can take her blood pressure. Her speaking continues to borderline abnormal as I pump up the BP cuff around her arm to about one-sixty and watch the needle hit at a real slow rate. So I send it up to one-eighty and it hits slow again. By now, Matt is standing with Derek and Ziffy, and the daughter is entertaining the three of them. Clearly showing now that she was amused by her mother's behavior. So I look over to Matt and I ask, "hey buddy, could you please set up a line for her?" I caught him off guard as he got serious and asked, "why?" "What's her blood pressure?" "I don't know yet, but we need a line and a strip," I said.

So Derek slid the monitor stickies above her breasts then one on each side. By now, I had pumped the cuff up to two-forty and it was still hitting. I finally got a pressure of two-eighty over one-forty with a rate of thirty-two, as the monitor showed a complete third degree heart block. I had only seen a couple of these before, but never with a pressure this high. And then it kicked in to me and I said to Matt, "she's been pacing herself all day," and I felt very enlightened. So I hit a line and Matt pushed a half-milligram of atropine. We both knew this wasn't going to work, it never does but its in the protocol. So we go through the motion before we set up the life pack to electrically pace our patient. As we sit her on the stairchair, we get capture on the monitor. Our patient's heart rate sets at eighty and she's going ow, ow, ow, ow. One ow each time a contraction captures. So we figure we can't bring her into the ER like this and we can't bring her in with a rate of thirty-two. So Matt suggests that we call for a sedation order and we get to push some morphine. Our patient had earlier suffered a big time heart attack, and they put a pacemaker in her right in the ER.

After the job we spoke about how we were caught off guard and even distracted by the patient's daughter. But all the same we had adjusted and didn't get burned. This particular job was educating, and showed me I could never really relax. We were back in service up on the triangle and I was thinking about telling Jason about this job in the morning along with our public porno stars at the bank. So we sit for about ten minutes then get to do a puking madman over by Edgecombe Park. A typical intoxicated weekend warrior, which killed about an hour of the tour.

As the night wound on, we continued to bang out the bullshit. At about six-thirty, we were woken for a cardiac arrest over in Mount Morris Park, by the pool. We got my buddy Mel and some rookie virgin named John backing us. I was buffing PD as we started rolling and we found out it was a shot. So we make some time getting over there and we arrive well before our backup. We drive the rig along the walking path into the park and head towards the red lights of the cop cars and the yellow tape. So we walk over towards the concrete stairs leading up to the pool. On the middle of the turning stairs is this guy in a pair of blue hospital scrubs, he's got an orange hospital ID bracelet on his wrist and nothing else. He's on his belly with his head turned to the side looking out. The man was shot once in the back of the head from point blank range with a three-fifty-seven magnum. This guy's got a large entrance wound and a spectacular exit wound out his nose. The whole front of his face was blown out and his nose was gone. Large chunks of brain matter were leaking out of the crater-like exit wound. And the flies were buzzing around in a feeding frenzy. So we're talking to the cops and I'm saying it looks like this guy might've escaped from the psycho ward or something and wandered down to the park. He probably started harassing the drug dealers in there and got capped.

By this time I was getting good at socializing at these scenes. As we continued to schmooze, Mel pulls up. His cherry partner comes flying out of the rig ahead of him carrying an oxygen bag and a BVM. It's a good thing he had to run about thirty yards to get to the body because I was able to pick him off before he made us all forget about Manny. I explained this was a crime scene and the guy was clearly a DOA. It took about ten seconds to sink in, but he turned around and brought the equipment back to the rig. As Mel and I showed him how to kill and hour doing paperwork, John thought I had been on the job about twelve to fifteen years by the way I handled this. And he made me laugh because he was such a baby buff. I said, "bro, I'm practically a rookie myself and just starting to get acknowledged around here as pond scum." And I explained how it seemed just like yesterday that I was just like him on a job with Tom.

We took the rig in for the change and Jason was waiting to start his day. I had a lot to tell him about and I was pretty burnt. I changed my uniform quick while Jason got the rig in service. When I got back up, he surprised me with coffee and ham and egg sandwiches. I was explaining that we had a typically fucked up night, but I felt like I had a lot of energy left. I had him laughing pretty hard, telling him about the ATM booth and it was real easy to keep him laughing describing John as robo-medic, running to bag brain matter. But we both agreed he was gonna be real good once Mel got him broke in and he understood the street culture a little better. So I'm continuing that this guy me and Matt were just on, was a really messy murder. One of our better ones I say. Then Jason responded that I was with him now and he felt like working hard. So I agreed to run with him and we buffed everything in site. I think we had already responded to twelve jobs in seven hours, when the big one hit about three in the afternoon, up on One–Four–Six between Broadway and Amsterdam.

We hear PD screaming into the radio for EMS that a guy hung himself off the fire escape in front of the building. Needless to say everyone and his mother was responding to this job. So it's assigned to 16–Victor with 16–Charlie on the back. Alex and Joey get on the scene first and they call out to come up the block the wrong way from Amsterdam because there's a lot of fire trucks and the cops blocking the street. So we pull up to living fucking insanity, its something right out of Steven King as this body is twirling in a brisk wind above a crowd of adrenaline juiced crazies. Everyone's got an opinion; everyone's got a story what happened. We get prepared to work right on the sidewalk as the firemen cut this guy down and the cops push our anticipating audience back and put up more of the familiar yellow tape. I can't help but be excited as I do my Raul Julia, "It's Show Time" voice, as the body comes down and Alex and Joey lay him supine on a board. I set up an 8.5 tube for this guy, and Jason was bagging for me as I did this and Alex began CPR.

As I'm getting ready to go in and I'm literally lying on my belly on the sidewalk looking down this guys oval of a trachea entrance. This cop comes running over to Jason hyperventilating and talking a mile a minute. He's grabbing his arm trying to pull him away saying, "come on, come on, she's upstairs, come on we need you upstairs." So I look up and I say point blank, "what the fuck do you think your doing?" And he tells us the scumbag that just did himself, stabbed his girl over fifty times before he jumped off the fire escape with a bed sheet tied around his neck. So Jason goes with the cop and a patrol supervisor up to the apartment. I look across at Joey and I blurt out, "go ahead pick your poison—traumatic arrest hanging or traumatic arrest stabbing." He said he would stay with me and his partner as I pushed the tube through the kinked windpipe right there on the sidewalk. A second BLS unit was on the scene now and we directed them upstairs telling them Jason was hung out up there. Some firemen helped us get our patient on the rig and he was a pretty big boy, only about thirty I thought. So Alex kept doing CPR and I let Joey dump a couple of epi's down the tube as I was right up next to him and pushed a fourteen gauge two-inch harpoon of and IV into this guys external jugular. Nothing like a good mid day hanging to create some JVD, I said as I ran the line open and flushed two more epi's, an atropine and just in case four milligrams of narcan straight down to the heart. Joey got up front and gave a notification to St. Luke's as to what we were bringing in. Alex worked like hell with me back there and units were waiting at the ER to help us get in, as I heard Jason and Jimmy giving a traumatic arrest notification to Harlem Hospital where they went with the girlfriend. When we came out of the ER about forty-five minutes later, the news vans had already set up camp outside the ER over on One–Twelve and Amsterdam. The chiefs and captains were enjoying the attention, and Alex and I headed to the station with Joey in the back to meet up with my partner. And then get the fuck out of there.

By the time we got done bullshitting, cleaning and restocking, my tour was getting close to eighteen and a half hours plus I still had a hour and a half ride home. I was telling Jimmy I don't think I can be back tonight and company man that he always was, he cut a deal with me so I could come in two hours late tonight. "Oh boy," I said excitedly as I left, "you mean I get a whole three hours sleep now?" The funny thing was, I was running on fumes, but I wasn't the slightest bit tired that night when I went back to start the whole fucking endless process again, only just a couple of hours later.

And Jimmy had kept the unit in service for the night, which kept me on his good side, which was very important to me.

Chapter 30

I've had a couple of pass days that allowed me to grow a few brain cells back. I pitched a tent in the backyard and built a picnic table out of two by fours. My daughters pretty much lived in the backyard with me as we practiced camping and they did surprisingly well—eating only barbecue and cooler food while sleeping in the tent all night with me, without a problem.

I get back on a cool Wednesday night. I've noticed the leaves are starting to change, so I'm looking forward to the ride home in the morning before I'm even in service. I hook up with Jason at the parking lot and he's bullshitting with the tour three party crew, while they kill a few beers. They were talking about our hanging/stabbing combo plate and another job that Jason did with Brendan while I was off. Jason filled me in that they had a guy who was a rigormortis DOA, stuck on top of a fence behind a building up on Wadsworth and One–Eight–Six. Apparently he was shot while fleeing someone, and he had two bullet holes in his back as he tried to go over a twelve-foot hurricane fence, lined along the top with a lot of prison type curling razor barbwire. Anyway, the guy never made it over and he was hung up there and had died while tangled in the mesh of razor wire along the top of the fence. I said, that's a once in a career job and even though he wasn't workable, I was ghoulishly disappointed that I missed it. We headed over to the station and he was happy to listen to my camping story as we got the rig in service, then headed down to One–Ten to get coffee and bagels. We're sitting down by Columbia University watching a few nice asses walk up Broadway and the radio suspects we might actually be enjoying ourselves.

We get an assignment way up town off of Audobon Avenue for an overdose. The text states, a fourteen-year-old girl took a bottle of pills. So we don't know if its bullshit or real and we need to cover over one hundred blocks uptown. We let Central know we'll be extended from One–Ten and Richie and Junior ask to back us up before we request. They get on the scene as we're approaching CPMC. Richie tells us that the girl swallowed a whole jar of aspirins, about a hundred and has been vomiting blood. Jason states the obvious to me that, "this isn't good," and we accelerate our pace further up Broadway. We get upstairs and the girl is in a lot of pain. She's crying and telling us, she's got a loud ringing in her ears, and there's a five-gallon bucket next to her bed with a lot of bloody vomit in it.

So it turns out this girl had been having a lot of emotional problems. I don't think she intended to really kill herself as much as she wanted attention. She was already packaged and ready to go down to the rig, as I asked Richie and Jason to get her downstairs while I called telemetry for a bicarb drip. It didn't take too long to convince the doctor of our need for this and when we got the kid over to CPMC, we looked pretty good to the nurses and doctor. Being that we didn't have a protocol for this but had been able to initiate the treatment needed, based on conveying a good over the phone history and having a definitive plan of action proposed.

So we got some more coffee over at the stick em up deli, and Richie and Jason were impressed at being able to obtain the drip order. Junior had no clue why we did this but we kinda got him up to speed on metabolic acidosis and you could tell Richie was starting to turn him into a good EMT. We went back into service as I finished my coffee and chain-smoked my third cigarette. We headed down to One–Three–Six on the triangle and waited for the radio to whip us again. You could hear the call volume starting to pick up and midnight madness was in full effect.

Earlier that afternoon a young woman checked herself into the emergency room at Harlem Hospital. She was very sick and thought she had a bad case of bronchitis. Well, she was admitted for pneumonia and later that evening was informed that she was HIV positive. Apparently, this was all she could take. She left the hospital AMA, then became our second job of the night. The dispatcher was in the process of assigning 11–Zebra an altered mental status, when she stuttered in mid sentence, "11–Zebra stand by." She then continued, "16–Victor, 13–Charlie, One–Three–Five and Lenox for the multi trauma in the subway." We were only one block up so as we responded I stated "6–Victor show me on the scene." We got down on the platform where we were informed by numerous witnesses, that a young-looking woman jumped in front of the train as it sped into the station. The train had passed over her completely and she was under the beginning of the fourth car. She had landed in the well between the tracks, and the first set of wheels to pass over her completed her self imposed execution instantly. The body was jammed up against a thick railroad tie while her head was totally separated from it about a foot further up, decapitated by a steel wheel of the Lexington Avenue Express cleaner than a guillotine. There wasn't too much to do other than paperwork for us. While Zif and Derek would be out of service two hours for a removal, and a trip down to the morgue. I had become pretty callous to these sights, and I don't believe that this job bothered me for too long, at least not consciously. But we quickly went in service and didn't talk about the job too much till later in the night.

I asked Jason to get us over to the bagel store for more coffee and chain-smoked four more cigarettes before we got another assignment. We get yo-yo'd back uptown again, on Pinehurst Avenue for a difficulty breathing. There's no back up available and again we're over a hundred blocks away. We have to cover Rich and Tom's area cause they're stuck on a hemorrhoid job down in Colonial Park. Either way it didn't matter, the way things were, everyone was getting banged and Central didn't give a fuck who was getting sent where, to do what.

We arrive on the scene in about ten minutes, which was actually pretty good response time and we got what appears to be a text book pulmonary edema in a large fifty-eight year old man. He's cold and wet, and you would think he just ran a couple of miles uphill the way he was breathing. We want to give nitros real quick, but I find out his BP is only 68/40 as Jason gives him oxygen and bangs out a strip of a-fib at one thirty. The guy is really shunted and neither of us can hit a line in the apartment. We wisely decide it's in everyone's best interest to start to get off the scene, being we have a three-flight carry down. All the guy's sons help us and we needed it. When we got down to the vehicle the patient's breathing was becoming slower and more labored, but he was still conscious. We were discussing if we should sit him up and risk bottoming him out or lay him down supine and risk drowning him in his own fluid. So we laid him on the stretcher half way in between. I got the BVM on him and Jason gave the Allen Pavilion a notification that we had a fifty-eight year old cardiogenic shock.

He took one more try at an IV telling me he was going to do one more stick then we were jettin'. He took an eighteen-gauge two-inch catheter and went two finger widths up and two finger widths out from the center crack of the inner forearm. Then he palped an area and inserted the needle far into the arm, hitting a deep brachial vein, and now giving the option of a fluid challenge or dopamine. This was a risky stick because it's not a superficial vein and it's close to the artery. But it was successful and that's what I believe mattered, as we started to roll with the patient, who was now very lethargic and his lungs were totally full. The BVM was becoming ineffective, as our patient was becoming a steel shade of gray and blue around the lips. I set up an 8.0 ET tube and then we approached the cobble stone street under the train. After making the patient supine, I asked Jason to slow down a little. As he did, I inserted a Mac 4 and quickly exposed the vocal chords. In less than five seconds I had the tube in place and attached to the BVM. Jason looked back and asked if everything was alright and I said, "yeah, he's intubated, keep going while I secure it." He gave me a thumbs up and we got into the ER about two and a half minutes later. And again had scored big time brownie points with the doctor.

We left knowing we would have an undocumented save. And I came to realize what I respected most now, was having people around me who knew what had to be done and weren't afraid to do it. I had come to live by this out here. Fear no job, do what needs to be done. It was gaining me a lot of respect but it was also gaining me some resentment and a few people used this against me, making me out to be a wildcard.

There was a happy medium in which the best medics thrived. But I was very emotional and passionate about my work and never really settled into that zone. And going out of my way to do what was right was ultimately going to be my demise. So after the job Jason is telling me he thought it was big balls for me to tube the guy alone, on the fly. I explained I didn't think so cause he was an imminent arrest and if I didn't clearly pierce the center of the chords on one try I was just gonna keep bagging him. So there really wasn't any risk and I said, "I didn't even know the vein you hit existed let alone where it was." I continued that I thought we made a real good team and that I wouldn't have tried to tube the guy with a lot of other partners. He said that he wouldn't have been able to go for that line with those same people. And I thought it was a shame that personalities and egos directly affected patient care.

The rest of the morning went along uneventfully. When we went in for the change, I bullshitted my way out of getting mandated. Then headed out of the city and up the Palisades. I lit up my version of the evening Martini, and slipped side three of Hot Rocks into the cassette player. Mick and Keith churned out Sympathy for the Devil as I thought the best part of this job was the ride out.

CHAPTER 31

I woke up today on less than three hours sleep. I had lined up a double with Jason and today was D-day, sixteen hours in the hood then I could rest a couple of nights. All I had to do was survive my double gauntlet. So it's a really shitty fall day, rainy, windy and very cold. At least being cold and wet will help keep me awake I thought. I took a quiet ride down to work and as soon as I stepped out of my car, I wound up in a three-inch deep puddle. My official hi-tech environmentally tested department issued boots had more holes than a block of Swiss cheese, so my spongy socks just about set my mood for me before I even got into the station. I was wet and tired and even just a slight bit cranky and assuming I didn't get banged with a late job. I only had sixteen hours and ten minutes to go before I could get out of this shithole.

We sign out our narcs and get the vehicle in shape for marathon bull-shit, knowing the recent nasty weather will assure us a multitude of congested dif breathers and allegedly unconscious flu patients. The Victor clinic/taxi service was open for business and business was brisk. So our first job out is a twenty-seven year old guy on One–Six–Three and Broadway. He's got a fever and tells us he's too sick to walk the five short blocks up to CPMC. Every time I have to climb the stairs or step into a makeshift piss pot for this kind of bullshit, my resentment grows a little larger. By this time the chip on my shoulder is only slightly smaller than a Buick, and as soon as my instincts and history tell me this guy is full of crap, I'm not talking anymore. I'm resigned to play car service and just end the assignment as soon as possible. So after getting the nurse to autograph my ACR, I mention to Jason "let's keep our ears open," this way we'll back up units and buff trauma or arrests and stay out of the flu loop. We're hanging out by the ER bay and we see Joey and Alex walking in another clinic job. We talk for a few minutes when they get out and we find out they both have been mandated till midnight, having started at eight in the morning. They're about as happy as me, and I let Alex know we're looking to stay away from bullshit. So, if anything sounds good don't worry about calling for a back.

We're listening to the PD radio hoping something will go down. If we go back in service, it's a sure thing we'll get hit with another dif breather. So we're stalling as long as possible when we hear 3–4–David, get sent out for a stabbing. A few seconds later the job comes over EMS and is assigned to 13–Charlie. So I get on the radio and I tell Central, "6–Victor is ninety-eight out of the ER, put us on Charlie's back." We get assigned to the job and head up to Two–O–Four off Tenth Avenue, reading the text that states a twenty-year old male has been stabbed and is in the lobby of the building. When we get on the scene, we find a guy in traumatic arrest. Apparently he had been with the wrong girl and was hacked with a machete by the jealous boyfriend. As I cut his clothes off Jason set up a tube for me. The patient had a long deep gash that was about ten inches and had cut right thru his clothes and even his ribs. It was one killing blow and extremely effective. Our backup arrived and the guy was put on a board. I began CPR, then quickly stopped as I noticed the top lobe of his lung came popping out of the wound with each compression. So I banged an 8.5 tube in and Jason dropped a fourteen in his upper forearm. We were off the scene in about six minutes and CPMC was notified we were coming hard with a young trauma arrest. When we got into the emergency room the doctor asked me to do CPR while they continued to work this guy up. I showed the physician how each compression brought the lung peeking out of the patient's chest cavity. It was at that time I learned that this was not a contra-indication to doing CPR, but I was too tired to feel stupid. When we were done, we both needed to go back to the station to shed wet, bloody shirts and restock the rig.

When we were ready to get back in service, it was around dinnertime. I saw Jimmy on the desk and he asked if I'd seen Sy lately. I hadn't and he said to me that he was in the hospital again with pneumonia. So I mentioned I would stop by in the morning to see how he was and then headed up to the triangle to wait out the rain, and our next assignment. So rain and MVA's go together like nachos and cheese and even allstatitis is better than three flight carry downs. We buffed a light damage motor vehicle accident and stayed busy with it for about an hour. We immobilized our theatrical neck and back pain patients and took them down to St. Luke's, where they would get the necessary paperwork to start the insurance claim that I'm sure a couple of years from now would pay off for them. I got us a couple of coffees from One–Ten and asked Jason if he could just infuse the caffeine into my veins via large bore IV. I had him laughing and he replied he could do it as a medical control option and would also request a French roast drip via piggyback. I was feeling pretty exhausted and was thinking I got twelve hours left. There's no light at the end of the tunnel yet, but I was about to get a big time, life changing adrenaline rush. That happened in a two minute span that I can replay in single frame time lapses. We were at the station bullshitting with Henry and Eugene; two old-timer, burnt out EMT's. The four of us are assigned a cardiac arrest on One–Two–Nine and Amsterdam. Jason and I head to our rig as Eugene starts bitchin' about working an arrest in the rain. "Calm down big guy," I'm saying to him. "It's probably some stiff eighty year old guy." "In twenty minutes, you'll be eating, while Jason and I do the paperwork." So no one read the text on the KDT, and when we arrived on the scene all hell was breaking loose.

I got out of the rig on the passenger side, while Jason got out on the street side and walked around the back of the vehicle to get the equipment from the rear, while I took our shit from the side. As Henry and Geno pull up behind us a fireman comes running out of the building holding a purple eighteen month old boy, followed by a couple of cops and a frantic, out of control mother. The woman was giving the kid a bath and left him alone to get a towel. When she got back to the tub, she said the boy was face down in the water. Well this lady was so freaked out; she couldn't bring herself to even touch the baby, being convinced she had caused his death. She was able to call 911 hysterically and the fireman said the kid was still face down in the bathtub when he arrived and the woman was on her knees screaming. Well they had initiated CPR but when I got him on the stretcher, he had no pulse or air movement. Henry jumped behind the wheel of our unit and we were off the scene in under a minute. I tubed the kid on the fly, while we sped down Amsterdam Avenue toward St. Luke's. I hit the tube easily and with no resistance as Jason said to me, "you got his life between your fingers, don't loose that tube", and he continued CPR. I looked over at him and the fireman who was in the back with me, and I angrily said, "this fucking kid is dead". I was listening to lung sounds as I continued to breathe for our baby. The tube is good, the tube is good, the tube is good, I mumbled this to myself with each squeeze of the BVM, as I heard air moving through the lungs.

Suddenly out of absolutely nothing, I heard a steady bup, bup, bup, bup, bup. The kid was in sinus tach after being a straight flat-line. I had a strong brachial pulse and his color went from purple to pink to normal in less than sixty seconds. When we were in the ER, the mother was on the verge of a nervous breakdown and in need of sedation. The nurses told her the baby was going to live and all she could do was cry while she ran to me and hugged me like clingwrap. When we left St. Luke's, Jason was electrified. He said that was the best clutch job he had ever seen, and my dick really was getting hard as it started to sink in just what had happened. For the time being, my manicness was on another all time high.

We went to get coffee and Jason was making my head as big as a beachball. He told me he was just getting the Broslow tape out and I already had the kid tubed. Then he asked how I knew what tube to use and which blade to go in with so quickly. I responded the kid was the same size as my daughter, and that I knew what I would do if it was my baby. I had instinctively put my plan of action to purposeful duty. He than continued that the reason the doctors had been asking me so many questions was because they were young guys who had spent a hundred thousand dollars on education, but had never done or seen a successful job like that. I really felt great as we left the store to get back on the vehicle.

We ran into Alex and Joey back at the station and another BLS crew of Manny-crime-scene and this dick Timmy who he had to work with. So I'm getting high praise from my partner and he's giving me all the credit, which is just the way he is. The guys are giving us much respect, but I see Timmy just giving me a jealous stare. We didn't get along and he was clear as glass to see through and phonier than the dope that the junkies shot through their veins. I thought of him as a mean, backstabbing, petty, bully, redneck, racist who, with diligence, had worked his way up to the status of station idiot. So when we leave, I'm talking with Jason and I say, "did you see Timmy's reaction when we were getting props?" I truly believe he's the kind of guy who would have enjoyed seeing me fail and the kid dying. Jason was too nice of a person to vocally agree with this, but his silence was a convincing acknowledgement of my ability to read scumbags.

We headed up to the triangle and in spite of being on the verge of emotional overload, I fell asleep deeply for ten minutes and when I woke it seemed like I was out for ten hours. We were headed uptown for a difficulty breathing, but we had a back, and we were eighty-seven'd before we even got to the scene, which I was very thankful for. The rest of the tour moved quickly as everyone we ran into gave us acknowledgement for the baby job. We rolled over at midnight, agreeing that a quiet rainy night was much needed. I spoke with Ziffy and Derek and later with Richie and Junior. I let them know that I was fried from working a double on no sleep and they agreed to eight-seven us off any bullshit and this was greatly appreciated.

It was after two in the morning when we heard 13–Charlie get a job off the George Washington Bridge for a MVA. We sat tight knowing that they wouldn't request medics unless it was absolutely necessary. They were on the scene approximately three or four minutes when Derek comes up on the air and asks Central, "status of 16–Victor." When dispatch informs him we're available he request medics and we're assigned to the job. This was the ultimate in respect and we made serious response time for them. When we get to their location, we find them off the exit ramp of the bridge, which corkscrews around and down to Riverside Drive. They got a DOA who was ejected from a Lexus. The guy was going really fast coming off the turn and he hit a dog while exiting the ramp. Then sideswiped into a two-hundred-year-old oak tree, which now occupied the spot that used to be the diver's seat.

Ziffy and Derek knew they had a DOA, and by requesting us, they figured we could make him an eighty-three and chill out for about an hour with them. These were the kind of favors I didn't forget. So after giving the doggie last rites, I lit a cigarette, took two puffs then placed it in between the lips of the mushed mutt. Jason told me I was a sick motherfucker and I nodded yes as I dragged my ass to the back of the rig and passed out on the stretcher for a half-hour, while the boys did the paperwork and rapped. After they packaged the corpse for his last ride. Jason woke me up and as the tow truck hooked up the Lexus. We went over to CPMC for coffee and I could finally see the light at the end of the tunnel. Thinking is my tour ending in a few hours or is it just the headlight of a train coming at me. I finished my coffee then went back to the deli and bought a can of soda called Jolt. It advertised double the caffeine and all the sugar, which sounded good to me. When I got on the vehicle, Jason asked me what it was that I was drinking and I responded, "instant pimple", as I handed him the can to sample and asked him to put us out of service facilities at hospital seventeen, so I could go sit on the bowl for a few minutes. I took off my boots and I contemplated my night, while on my throne. My socks were still soaked and my toes were resembling big pale raisins. I let myself air out a little, then went back to the rig and got back into the flow of things. We put ourselves back in service and laid low until sunrise. By now I was so tired my head was tingling and I was hearing a buzzing noise as I struggled to stay awake. We finished our tour with Richie and Junior backing us up on an early morning overdose on One–Eight–One and Fort Washington in the street.

They arrived on the scene first and the patient was already packaged and on their stretcher as we pulled up. So I got in the back of the rig with Jason, and Junior drove our vehicle while Richie taxied us down to CPMC. Jason was really tired too, but I was wiped out. This guy was moving good air and neither of us were in the mood for puke or stupidity. So we rode to the hospital, monitoring our failed street pharmacist. As we backed into the ER bay, I banged two milligrams of narcan right thru his pants and into his ass cheek. We presented him as an OD without venous access and as he started to wake up, he became their problem. I told the triage nurse that we had given him narcan IM and we were out of there quickly and back for the change with out getting whipped again.

I was totally wiped out and hoping I didn't crash my car again due to fatigue and I still needed to go see Sy. So he was up on the eighth floor at Harlem hospital, and when I got up there my metabolism was burning so fast that I was sweating like a shanked pig, even though it was like thirty-five degrees out. I walk into his room and he's happy to see me. I say to him, "will you just fucking get better already or die," and to my shock Sy replied, "dude, I got the big one." I was still kinda in denial and I should of figured out what was wrong with all his pneumonia's. So I say, "get the fuck out of here, your just fucking with me, right?" "No," he said, "I got HIV." My heart sank, I really hated this disease and I wouldn't wish it on my worst enemy, let alone my best friend. I felt very emotional as I said, "I sincerely wish I was smarter so I could do something about this fucking miserable sickness." Sy knew how tired I was and he appreciated me coming by. Before I left I went down to McDonalds and smuggled a breakfast up to him, so at least he didn't have to eat the cardboard that the hospital called food.

When I drove home, the whole night and a few other jobs were flashing through my head, invading what little sanity I had left. I listened to Pink

Floyd, Welcome to the Machine, and chain-smoked almost a whole pack of cigarettes, while tears involuntary flowed down my cheeks. I needed a break real bad and three nights off wasn't going to be enough, as I continued to endure the whole fucking endless process.

CHAPTER 32

I'm back at work but I don't want to be here anymore. The pride in my unit and my true partners will always be there, but the constant political bureaucracy has worn me down, along with the personality clashes, the commuting, the never ending mandates, conflicting child care, and constant flow of job after job that's not worthy of a Band-Aid, let alone an emergency response. When we get real jobs they usually end in repetitive concentrated misery and it always seems like the meaningful work is completely covered under a pile of steaming dogshit. I know that 99% of everything that happens is bullshit, and 99% of what's left I don't even remember twenty minutes after it happens.

I've come to realize that I can have all the good intentions in the world and be on top of my game for twenty-three hours and fifty-nine minutes. But if I relax and let my guard down for one minute, that's the minute everyone will talk about and remember. So I'm just going about my life. I think I really let everything get to me and tried to hide behind sex, reefer and alcohol. So another thing I've come to realize is that it's also a full time job just being a decent human being. Wake up, do your thing, don't fuck anyone. Be a good person, survive and advance. Most people can't even be bothered with this and the simple equation remains a timeless mystery. I'm ruled by my emotions. This sucks. I only wanted to try to make good, but I got stomped again. I remind myself that good days need to be created not expected, but this battle which should never be has worn on me also.

So I'm on the rig with Brendan and in spite of the good things we had been doing, he knew I was way off my game tonight. He covered my slack and didn't make a big deal out of it, which I appreciated. I didn't want to tell him I was on daily antidepressants that weren't working. And at that time I couldn't give an honest answer to what I was feeling. So our night dragged on and in the morning, I knew we would be working again tonight. As I left, I apologized for not being great company and said I was gonna do some fall planting today and shake off the blahs, as he replied just feel better and be careful driving.

I did a lot of bulb planting that morning and didn't sleep well during the afternoon. When my alarm clock went off at nine-thirty, I was in a coma and even cold water couldn't remove the crust from my eyes. The drive down was quiet time for me and as I got closer and closer to the bridge my stomach tightened up, as feelings of dread bombarded me. When I got to the station, I was determined to be a good guy and fun partner. I would be able to pull this off for eight hours, the problem was I would bring the shit home with me now and I was turning into a real douchebag with my wife.

So were working on 13–Willie tonight and it's the day before Halloween. Which really doesn't mean anything up here, but that's just what day it was. Our night starts out with a pediatric upper respiratory infection, which is good and bad. It's no stress and an hour closer to the end of our tour, but I hate being used as a taxi and this makes my stomach bubble. We reach a compromise on food after the job and we agree. I won't get an onion bagel with lox and cream cheese, if Brendan won't eat the extra greasy super spicy chicken wings with death sauce. So we go get Chinese food through the bullet proof glass, then head over to the graveyard to try to eat before the streets catch up with us. I'm sitting on the passenger side of the rig staring at the weathered and chipped tombstones. Some of which are from the 1750's and are completely blackened from age and New York air. As I continue to peer through the black wrought iron gates, the radio gives us an assignment over on One–Seven–Three and Audobon for a trauma. The text is only stating that we have a male bleeding at the scene and we're both happy to find out it's a street job.

When we arrive at the corner a large crowd has gathered and is mostly people costumed from a party at a club over there. So we grab our shit off the bus and we can see a large, shattered plate glass window, where our patient was ejected from the Halloween party. This guy is laying on the sidewalk dressed like a Hula girl, he's got it all goin' with the grass skirt, loud shirt and a lei along with lots of flowers in his hair. As cute as he looked he had a couple of major immediate problems, one of which was a huge gash on his inner forearm that was bleeding profusely. So we load him into the rig and he's clearly intoxicated. Slurring and almost knocking me out with his blowtorch breath. Brendan bangs a fourteen gauge IV and I'm getting good pressure on the wound as the bleeding is now pretty much under control. But while I'm adjusting the oxygen mask, I notice a lot of blood staining the stretcher sheet around where his ass is. I ask Brendan if he saw any other lacerations. He replied "heads or tails," as we both knew one of us needed to examine under the grass tutu. So being that Brendan was closer, I suggested that fate had already determined that he check the genitalia. Sure enough the guy's underwear are blood-soaked and we didn't think this Hula gal had his period. So Brendan cuts off his briefs and as he lifts a half severed penis he says to me, "well I hope he had his kids already."

The guy's dick was still connected but it was cut bad, right at the base above his nut sack. So yes we made all the Lorena Bobbitt jokes and when Brendan told me he was driving, I asked, "but I thought you we're gonna apply direct pressure…with your tongue." We gave CPMC a notification, but didn't mention the extent of the injuries over the air. Our guy was so bombed he didn't realize he was gonna need some serious reconstructive surgery. When we got into the emergency room, he was quickly sedated by the doctor. So after the staff gets finished making all the same jokes we did ten minutes ago, we walk out into the ambulance bay and while Brendan goes and gets us coffee, I'm standing there smoking a Marlboro and I can't get the song "Detachable Penis" out of my head.

The night moves on and we do the taxi-shuttle-clinic thing for a few hours with a puking madman thrown in. When at about five-thirty the dispatcher lets us know we have a trauma on the FDR Drive, PD is calling for a rush, which means this is a real job considering it's not close to their tour change. Ziffy and Derek are backing us up and the voice on the other end of the radio is talking very fast, telling us the cops got a guy with his leg severed on the southbound approach, on the steep hill that exits from the bridge. Brendan lights up the rig and makes ludicrous speed over to the scene. We arrive to find a bad news, worse news job. The bad news was this guy was coming across the George Washington when he got a flat on the front drivers side tire. The worse news was that while changing that flat tire, someone came speeding around the turn and down the hill, severing his leg above the knee and twisting it back out of his hipsocket.

Once again we didn't have a complete separation of limb from his body, but his femur was crushed pretty good from the impact of a car passing over it at high speed. And this guy's leg looked like chopped meat that was pounded out with a baseball bat. This patient needed to get down to Bellevue pronto. Much to my surprise there wasn't an unreal amount of bleeding and there wasn't much I could do in regard to stabilization of the leg, as our rig flew down to the replantation facility. When we were done with the job, the sun was up and shining. We headed uptown after doing our restock and decon over at Station 13. We snuck back into our area via the barrio. It was literally two minutes till the tour change when Central bent us over for another one of those, now I've seen everything jobs.

"13–Willie," the radio calls. We both look at each other as neither of us will pick up the mic, hoping our sadistic voice of gloom will just keel over or something. So it continues, "13–Willie, sorry guys I need you for one more." I answer the gnawing summons, "Willie go." "One–One–Nine and Lexington for an unconscious at that location," we're told. So both of us are pretty tired but since we're getting a job anyway, we figure we'll juice this one good for the time and a half. When we get on the scene

Central asks us to let her know if we have a patient or not and I respond I will, as soon as I get done with my daily morning stair climbing workout. So we get all the way up to a sixth floor apartment that was being rented to a sixteen year old girl. She was recently on her own and experiencing a lot of problems handling her new found freedom. So Brendan asks her what the problem is and she tells us her cat is unconscious. As I pick my jaw up off the floor, she continues that her cat is a diabetic and is supposed to get insulin twice a day but she didn't have any.

Sure enough we have a feline coma at the scene and neither one of us really knows what the fuck to do with this. So I get on the air and request a patrol supervisor. Central asks if we have a patient at the scene, before granting our request. I say not exactly, but we have a problem here that we would like some help with. So Central asks again in that really snotty obnoxious voice, "13–Willie, do you or do you not have a patient at that scene?" I respond "I got an unconscious tabby." "Can I please have a patrol boss." We could see this kid was really stressed out and didn't know what to do for her pet. I felt bad for her and so did Brendan. I told her, "I'll get some help for you, but I need to talk with my boss first." So Jimmy is out on patrol today and I'm glad the law of averages didn't prevail by sending us a douchebag like Lieutenant Lardass or Lieutenant Handjob. I tell Brendan there's an animal hospital down on the river at Sixty-ninth Street and maybe Jimmy will let us give her a ride down there. Well when he shows up, I got this cat on oxygen and he's explaining to this girl how we can't do anything for animals.

Well being we were on overtime as it was, we would never be allowed to take a pet to the veterinarian, in addition to all the health code violations this would have involved. So Jimmy eighty-seven'd us and told us to get home safe, then he gave the kid and her cat a ride down to the animal hospital in the patrol vehicle, and I actually felt good for a few minutes that morning. When I drove home I thought more about the girl and her cat than I did about all the shit that was upsetting my karma and making me crazy.

CHAPTER 33

The day opens up as I'm riding down the Palisades to work a double with Jason, sixteen hours in the hole. I'm still seeing the wonderful fall colors on the trees and I'm listening to California Dreaming. I'm deeply in the fantasy of leaving, as I continue my ride and the world goes on around me.

About this time fifty miles south of my location, an old man is shopping with his wife at the mall in Patterson, New Jersey. When they come back to their Mercedes, some junkie and his girlfriend are waiting. They stick a 9mm in the women's face and demand the keys to the car. This is happening in the middle of the afternoon and in the parking lot where many witnesses are present. One of which, is an armed private security guard. So the owner of the car quickly cooperates with the demands of the car jackers and in spite of this, his wife is still pistol-whipped and left lying on the ground bleeding badly. As the vehicle speeds out of the parking lot, the guard sees an opportunity for a clear shot and pumps five rounds into the back of the car blowing out the rear window as it turns out onto the highway and accelerates away. At this time for me, the Mommas and Pappas are playing Go Where You Wanna Go, and I continue my ride, mentally wandering in a flood of orange, gold and red foliage, not knowing what the day holds for me and at that time not really caring either.

An hour or so later, I'm in service on 16–Victor with my favorite partner. I'm trying to cheer him up a little which in itself is role reversal. Jason had worked with Tom a couple of nights ago and they had a tough tour that ended with a late job under the Cross Bronx Expressway. They were assigned a traumatic arrest and it turned out to be a rape all the way down in the weeds. It was actually under the FDR Drive and the approach from the bridge. Jason went on to tell me they walked almost a half a mile down the winding bushy paths, before they found an unconscious thirty-two year old woman down by the waterline of the Harlem River. She had been beaten so bad that you couldn't tell if she was a male or female till you got close. There was dirt all over her body and mud on her face and caked into her teeth from having her head pushed down into it. The woman also had extensive trauma to and around her vaginal area. And this wound up being a really difficult job for him to blow off and move on from.

So I'm saying things to the effect of "I really need you to get happy, we both can't be manic or else the wheels will really be off the unit." So I got him to crack a smile, but I could tell Jason was having a bad day and it was just starting. We continued to talk and I let him vent off some steam, as the radio called and continued the mental and physical assault that seemed endless at best. "Six Victor" it called out. "Victor go," I responded. "One–Seven–Eight and Broadway for the trauma." I hit the six-three button, lit up the bus and called up the job on the KDT. This assignment is right on the ramp coming off the bridge next to the Port Authority, and the text is stating that there's a woman in a car bleeding at the scene. So we both figure we have a car accident and I'm hoping its bullshit cause neither of us is into an immobilization and transport at this time.

We pull up the ramp going against traffic and parallel park next to a sharp looking black Mercedes 560 SEL. It takes about half a second to see the girl in the front passenger seat slumped off to the side against the door and shattered glass all over the back seat. As I checked the woman for responsiveness and a pulse, a sense a numbness comes over me as the familiar feel of death covers my senses. The woman has a huge gunshot wound in the back of her head with no exit. Apparently this was the vehicle that was car jacked in Patterson a couple of hours earlier. The guard who fired on it was probably aiming for the driver, but he wound up capping the girl instead.

Her scum bag lowlife boyfriend, drove up to the city then as soon as he crossed the bridge, abandoned the car and her body, leaving them both parked right on the ramp. We figured she died instantly, but probably continued to bleed for about a half-hour before this asshole figured out that he just got his girl perished. We let Central know that we had an eighty-three and a crime scene, true to my word. I did the paperwork for this and we moved on to the next victim. By now I've become hardened enough to expect anything but we got an assignment over on One–Four–Seven and Bradhurst that surprised me, not so much the job itself but what caused it and how it unfolded.

The address we were going to didn't exist. Most of the buildings around there were just burnt out shells so you couldn't exactly tell what the number was prior to its infernoization. So we finally figure out where it is we're going to and this place is a hub of activity with squatters, whores and drug users. One of the things that goes on in this place is dogfights and some of these people bet large amounts of cash on their animals. Anyway, this particular fight matched a kick ass, nasty pitbull against a collie. Well everyone who hears about this fight thinks it's easy money. This sucker is gonna get his lassie dog killed in about thirty seconds, then get himself cleaned out. But this is no cutie pie lassie doggy, this collie is about a hundred and sixty pounds and is mangy as all hell, having never been cleaned and for the last five years eating gun powder mixed into it's food.

Well this fucking animal was seriously bad news. When they let the dogs go on each other, the pit immediately latched onto the collie's throat and locked down, but the stupid motherfucker had nothing but a mouth of fluff as it couldn't penetrate deep enough to make contact with flesh. In about ten seconds the collie with its long sleek jaws, came under the pitbull while it was still locked on fur. It ripped the other dog's belly completely opened, leaving the pitbull whimpering in a puddle of blood with its intestines hanging out, resembling Italian sausage or kielbasa. The pit's owner was shocked and just a little pissed off. Apparently he freaked out and slashed the collie's owner across his face with a straight razor. The person who got slashed in turn, pulled out a thirty-two caliber semi auto and squeezed off four shots into the other guy's chest. So as we walk onto the scene with PD, I'm barely moved as I stepped around the dead dog. But I have to admit, I too would've bet on it. We had Junior and Richie on our back and had to split up. My slashing guy really wasn't to bad except for the fact that after he got stitched up, he was gonna get old in Elmira. So I grabbed Junior and we shuttled down to St. Luke's with the cop on board and our patient handcuffed to the stretcher. Richie and Jason took the imminent arrest to Harlem and we met up back at the station an hour or so later. So at least this calamity got Jason's mind off of his recent rape job and we bullshitted about it for about half an hour before the trauma hawks needed to transform back to the yellow cab company for a few hours.

The weather was starting to turn again and if nothing good was going down we were sure to stay busy with the usual sniffle/dif breather and congestion/chest pain. Anyway the rest of the tour can't keep up with beginning and at midnight. I go change into a clean Batman suit and roll out for another round as Harlem's whore. We got into service and headed up to St. Nick to sit on the triangle. The EMS god was feeling benevolent as we had been in service a whole fifteen minutes and hadn't gotten a job yet. So we decided to take advantage of the lull and head over to white castle for some brick burgers and wood chips. I get some food for us and say no to the crackhead outside the place who asks me for some change as I walk back to the rig. So I'm my normal self or at least close to it and Jason seems to have shaken off his rut. Naturally I'm breathing so I must be bitching this time it's about the food as I'm ranting "I don't know why I eat this shit." "I should just order a Coronary Artery Disease with cheese." "Man, I got indigestion just looking at it and I'll probably have the runs all day." This loosened up Jason good and I had him laughing pretty hard. When Ziffy came up on the radio and asked Central, "status of 16–Victor," dispatch answered that we were available for an assignment and he then requested medics.

So we don't know what they got, being they were sent to an unknown condition all the way up on Cabrini Blvd. and we were way down on One–Two–Five and Powell. So we jump on the Henry Hudson Parkway at One–Three–Two and give them a seven-minute ETA. When we arrive they're in a ground floor apartment. Yes, an actual lobby apartment. No walk up, no vertical urinal, what a concept. Anyway, Derek meets us at the door and he tells me our patient is Casper. So I'm looking at him a little funny and when we get into the living room, there's wet white paint everywhere and a huge puddle with an empty five-gallon bucket in the middle of it.

We go into the bedroom and find a young girl who had been involved with some kinky sex that went too far. She's sitting on the edge of the bed kinda dazed out like she's on ecstasy or something, and she's talking to Zif and the cops. Her boyfriend had painted every inch of her body with white latex paint, then got pissed off and dumped the rest of the bucket over her head. She locked herself in the bedroom after he started beating on her, and tried to climb out the window. She was pretty slimy and slipped through the glass out onto the sidewalk, where Derek and Zif found her naked and bleeding. The cops got there about the same time as them and took her back into the apartment, but the boyfriend was already gone, leaving white footprints out of the building and up towards the Cloisters. The broken glass that resulted from her escape sliced deeply into her arms and thighs. Even though Ziffy and Derek had somewhat cleaned her up and put a sweatshirt on her, she was still covered with paint and blood. I thought she was artistically bizarre, as we continued to try to contain the source of the jagged red streams that ran down her milky white body. The girl was transported over to the Allen Pavilion and Joanie the triage nurse asked us if she had been auditioning for the pure and natural Ivory girl commercial. I commenced with the longwinded details while Ziffy filled in the remainder of the story. When we left the hospital, I used my never underestimate the power of a good history line, then threw another failed dinner to the pigeons.

The rest of the night dragged on with a bunch of bullshit jobs that would lead you to believe the side of our bus read Abuse Me, and not FDNY * EMS. When the night ended, I was pretty tired but I decided I still had enough energy to go find one of hardcore smoking buddies, and have the breakfast of champions...a bone of hydros.

Afterwards I headed up the Deegan as a change of pace, just to cruise over the Tappanzee Bridge. When I got home, I played some Nintendo with my daughter and the next thing I knew I was being woke up from the couch at nine thirty, still in my uniform. It was time to get changed and start the whole fucking endless process again.

CHAPTER 34

I wake to November Rain invading my peace, static-ing through my clock radio. I've been sleeping five hours but it feels more like five minutes as my eyes are glued together with drowsy crust. I'm not in the mood to wake up but I need to continue the whole fucking endless process to pay my bills. So I drag my lazy ass out of a warm bed that has me covered in about seven heavy down comforters. I start my car as my breath frosts out my nostrils. The holiday season is coming again and although I'm thankful for what I have, I'm still feeling like I got penance to do, as I head down the thruway to meet up with Matt for another round of hell meets reality. Matt got mandated today for six, so he's pretty fucking cranky and his baby face is a little rustled as he hadn't had a chance to shave today, yesterday or the day before.

We go into service as Cinderella's coach turns into a pumpkin, and Central inflicts tonight's version of operation mind crime. Porkchop, the dispatcher, gives us a job at twelve-o-one with her mouth filled with jelly donuts. 16–Victor, she gags, are you in service yet? "Not presently," Matt responds. Well its twelve-o-two and we literally just signed out our narcs and haven't even put the key in the vehicle yet. So Porky responds, "16–Victor you have an assignment, One–Eighteen and Lexington for the trauma." "Fucking piece of fucking shit." I'm ranting "fuck you, you fat do nothing waste of sperm bastard." I tell Central in my most polite appreciative manner, "OK send the job and mark me six-three, unchecked vehicle." So we head over to the scene and we don't call up the job, neither of us really gives a shit what we got. A job is a job and at this point who cares if it's a traumatic arrest or a bleeding hemorrhoid, we'll just fucking bang it out, then bang out ten more for the lowly scrupples, these political assholes call a paycheck. We head over to One–Eighteen and when we arrive the cops are standing over this guy whose on the sidewalk resembling a frog. This unfortunate soul had been involved with someone else's wife, but the husband was wise to the play. He left for the night, then came back home with bad intentions. He had a few of his boys with him and when he let them in the apartment with him, Romeo and Juliet we're moaning the song of lust.

So what happened next was, this naked second-hand gigolo was trying to get to the door, when he got the beat down of his life. After kicking the shit out of him, they decided he should leave via the fourth floor window, but Romeo didn't leave easy. He clung to the window's edges and dug into the sides like a cat on a doberman's back. While the husband was trying to kick him out the window one of the other guys got a carving knife and was stabbing him in the chest, hands, and arms trying to accelerate, the flying process. When Romeo finally flew he crash-landed on the sidewalk below and became my first job of the chilly night. He laid on the sidewalk with multiple stab wounds, extensive body wide trauma and a couple of broken arms, that were bent up and back in an unnatural way. So our patient isn't dead at this time, but he's not gonna be in this world much longer. He's totally unconscious and has shallow rapid respirations.

So while we're working on this guy, the cops are busy arresting the husband and to this day, I still don't know who had the more fucked job, us or the police as this guy was totally psycho. Anyway the patient that Matt and I are dealing with, landed like a swan dive on his hands and head. He was clamped up really tight and I had a hard time getting an oral airway in him. I figured since we don't carry any paralytics with us, I'm not gonna add to the patients problem by breaking his teeth trying to intubate him.

So I bag the guy all the way over to St. Luke's, after Matt dropped a couple of lines in him. The ER staff would have a much easier time securing his airway further, after we arrived, than we would've had try-ing to fight the tube in on the bus. It really was all for show because this person would end up being stiff and on the slab before my tour was done. So fortunately for us tour three left the rig in good shape. So even though we were unchecked, we didn't get burned. After the job we put ourselves out of service, decon and restock, and got to pick up bagels and Java before heading back to the station.

The night seemed longer than usual and we were making small talk about some medics in Brooklyn who were gonna get roasted for being involved in a morphine scandal. Apparently they got caught popping holes through the tops of the vials and drawing out the narcotic, then replacing it with normal saline and keeping the dope for themselves. Matt was saying how this would never happen in Harlem and that the station had never had a problem involving the controlled substances. I replied back, "yeah that's just because we can get better shit right around the corner." Besides, EMS dope would probably just make you sick. So I had Matt smiling as we continued to bullshit, then picked up a seizure job for Tom and Rich up on Seaman Avenue. We finished our morning over on One–Four–Five and Lenox with a woman who had been mugged while entering the subway to go to work. She wasn't busted up or anything, but she was extremely agitated and shaken from her ordeal. But the reality was, she was more of a PD job than an EMS job. She did want to go to the hospital to get checked further and her pressure was kinda elevated, which was no surprise.

Anyway we got off on time, while PD did their report from the emer-gency room. I parked the rig and turned in my paperwork. After I said goodbye and get home safe to Matt, I got the fuck out of there before the sky fell and I didn't get mandated. I couldn't leave fast enough and all I really wanted to do now was smoke a fat one while I watched sports center. Then fall asleep, so I can spend some time with my kids in the afternoon, before I had to go back that night to work with Jason and you know something about an endless fucking process.

CHAPTER 35

So the beginning of the end for me starts like any other day. I wake up with a stomachache and pop a couple of zantacs. The shower doesn't do much to improve my immediate alertness, and I grab a cold chicken cutlet out of the fridge, and eat it with my hands as I warm up my car and try to wake up a little more by blasting Iron Maiden. I get to work about fifteen minutes late and Jason already has the rig ready for the grind. As I arrive and put my shit on the vehicle. It's been kinda rainy and shitty all day. So when we get into service, I suggest some coffee, then go park by the river and listen to the water till we get a job. We've been hanging out now about fifteen minutes, which is about as long as we can go without an assignment. Central must sense we're comfortable, so they pick a beauty for us. "16–Victor, One–Four–O and Hamilton Place for the EDP," the radio breaks in. Jason responds that we're six-three and we head over to the location.

When we pull up we find this Spanish guy running up and down the block with a crab net catching pigeons about two or three at a time and stuffing them into a laundry bag. So I approach this guy with cautious optimism and cheerfully ask, "excuse me my man, how are you tonight?" The guy looks at me and quick a cat, he bags another pigeon as he replies, "I'm fine, what can I do for you?" So now Jason is with me and he says someone called 911 cause they thought maybe you needed some help. So we were both pretty taken by this guy. He was very personable and made it clear that he preferred to eat these flying rats, even after we offered to buy him some fried chicken and fries. So I ask Jason should we make him a ninety or ninety-three? We decide to just make him a ninety and let Central know we don't have a patient at this location. The guy catches two more pigeons then goes into a building on the block, as we wave goodbye to Col. Sanchez and leave the area. So the night moves on and a couple of hours later we're dispatched to an MVA with 13–Charlie up on Broadway near Dyckeman. There's a pretty sharp curve right before that intersection, and we arrive simultaneously with Derek and Ziffy to find an eighteen-wheeler has gone head on with a convertible.

So the firemen are on the scene first and they already got a twenty-four year old guy out of the vehicle and sitting on the curb wearing a cervical collar that's up around his nose (this is not exactly protocol). So the first thing you notice is the engine block is in the ashtray and this was another one of those how the fuck did he survive jobs. I start to walk towards the patient with Jason while Ziffy and Derek grab a board and the stretcher off their rig. So this yokel hose-head is saying how the patient is OK, and he probably just needs an x-ray, as we get close enough to see the patient sitting there having a seizure. So now we accelerate our patient care and degree of seriousness. As Jason gets off the telemetry unit with a valium order, I have a sixteen in place. The fireman still doesn't know what the fuck is going on yet and as I intubate our now comatose patient I think he starts to realize they fucked up. We get off the scene soon afterwards and notify CPMC of our approach. The kid wound up having a bad bleed into his brain and was another miserable ending.

At about three-thirty, 12–Young gets a job for a difficulty breathing on One–Two–Seven and Lenox. They're whining over the air about how they're extended from Nine–Six and Two, and asking for a BLS backup to respond first and give them an update. Well no one is backing these skells and no one is making themselves available either. So I ask Jason, being that we are closer anyway, if he wants to pick up the job so these pudknockers can go get a diaper change. We inform Central we're right in that area and volunteer for the assignment.

We arrive to find a fifty-three year old female in full blown pulmonary edema. She's so full she can't even speak and as I lightly touch her cheek with the back of my hand I know she's real by the cold wet feel. So I ask Jason to give me the nitros and I want to get a BP quick so we can give them. I never get the chance, as I'm pumping up the cuff around her bicep, she slumps forward and arrests right into my arms. So the family has no clue what's going on and the daughter is still telling us the patient must go to St. Luke's, cause that's where her records are. We get her on the floor supine and Jason begins CPR. Then he informs the daughter we must go to the nearest hospital now which is Harlem, as I get on the air and request a backup forthwith for a witnessed cardiac arrest.

Ziffy and Derek responded from One–Six–Six and Amsterdam and flew downtown to meet us. Henry and Eddy also volunteered to back us and before we knew it we had more competent help than needed. While still in the apartment I bang a 7.5 tube while Jason misses three shots at a line. This woman's got nothing. She's so shunted and overweight I can't even palp an external jugular. On top of that she's a diabetic too and we can't even find a vein in her feet. So I'm trying to breathe for her and the positive pressure of the oxygen being pushed into her lungs is bringing all this bloody fluid up the tube. I try to push an epi in, but it just foams out the top of the tube like a champagne bottle that's just been popped. So we get her packaged and down to the rig. While we're coming down the stairs I tell Jason I'm going IJ on her in the vehicle. "You're the man Dano, do what you gotta do," he replied.

Jason jumped in the back with me and Eddy was back there too as Henry drove. I felt like a kernel of popcorn in the popping machine as we took off down the pothole marred Ho Chi Min trail known as Lenox Avenue. Our patient was still flat-line as I pulled a harpoon of an IV from my belt pouch. I gave Eddy control of the ET tube and then went into the patient's neck at a forty-five degree angle right over the clavicle and into the internal jugular with a fourteen-gauge two-inch IV. As the maroon blood shot up the catheter I knew my hit was good, and quickly pushed an atropine and epinephrine through the line and straight down to the heart. As we backed up to the ambulance bay our patient was in sinus tach and had a strong carotid pulse.

So what happens next is living proof that any idiot who can occupy a seat for six years can be a doctor. This big fat moron female doctor tells me this is a central line. So I nodded yes. Then she tells me I'm not authorized to do central lines under my certification and that this is a very invasive procedure. Which is true, but at this time we have a save and not a corpse, which I feel is all that mattered. Anyway after the patient is stabilized and a chest x-ray confirms my line to be good, this fat bastard is still giving me a hard time. So I sarcastically pointed out that my options were limited to lividity or rigormortis and the fact that the patient was clearly flat-line and now alive showed I wasn't pushing drugs into a collapsed lung.

So I left and Jason did the paperwork trying to cover me by documenting I had started an external jugular and not a central line. About twenty minutes later, Lieutenant Lardass puts us out of service, administrative procedures, and we get patient care restricted. So there's no way in hell I'm letting my partner hang for this too. I'm going absolutely fucking ballistic and I'm saying we volunteered for the job. We didn't even have to fucking be there, we could've just let 12–Young take their sweet ass time getting to a job they were assigned to and the patient would've just been dead when they got there. The bottom line is that I did what was needed and appropriate for the patient and went above and beyond to try to save a life. Then I swore up and down that my partner had no idea what I did. It was my decision solely to initiate a central line and he thought it was just an EJ and documented it as so. Then I put that statement in writing and got Jason off the hook. But this was just what my detractors had been waiting for. My reward for trying to preserve life was I would get full medic pay to stand around the station with my thumb up my ass and watch my unit go down the shitter. While scrubbing long boards and shuffling paper till I got fed up enough to quit. It was hard to discipline me on this issue because on merit we were right. But the department is more concerned with liability and public image then patient care, and some of the douchebags I pissed off had me by the nuts.

My supporters told me they knew I did well, but if I was rewarded other medics might also attempt this and people would be dropping lungs all over the city. My detractors countered with, I was an out of control wildcard, and what was next, chest tubes on a shooting, surgical crychs on an obstruction?

Anyway I thought the press would be interested in knowing how you save a life and get fucked over, while continuing to get paid to do nothing while people wait twenty minutes for an ambulance. Anyway I think the higher ups knew I would e-mail this story to every media person within five hundred miles. So no one really bothered me and I was left hanging in limbo, while Jason's reward was he got to work with some skeevy transvestite who was inserted into my slot. And everyone in the city knew he was getting fucked too, probably for no other reason than his loyalty to me. So after playing maid around the station for a few days I found myself renewing my antidepressant prescription.

When I got to work that night I knew something was terribly wrong immediately. Sy looked lost and people all around the base were crying. I found out one of the guys we work with had been killed that night by a cop car speeding after a suspect. I was very tight with this man, and took this very hard. While talking about it with Sy, we felt the story given was really suspicious and that had one of us killed a cop by accident with the ambulance, we would be super sizing orders if we ever got out of prison.

So anyway it was about this time that everything was boiling over on me. I was hair triggered and looking for a victim when someone presented himself for sacrifice. This little Barney Rubble clone, a real nasty scumbag had been fucking with me from day one. I had been walking away, turning the other cheek and all that other happy bullshit, but today was the last straw. Well this piece of shit really was a professional button pushing blowjob and after the funeral was acting stupid and getting all personal with me at the restaurant. It was if like when Popeye says "that's all I can stands, I can't stands no more."

I got close to Barney and said, "you're a fucking jerk off," as I hit him with the greatest left hook that I ever threw in my life. Starting it down around my ankles and crashing my fist full bore with everything I had into his face. I knocked him clean over the table and in that split one tenth of a second, I felt better then I had at anytime in the last few weeks. So I knew this was gonna get broken up fast and I also knew I had just committed occupational suicide, so I was getting as much mileage as possible out of this. I got to him on the other side of the table and helped him up by his throat. I consciously said to myself, OK be fast, turn it into a hockey fight. I then held him with my right and fired about thirty short lefts in ten seconds, connecting solidly with all of them. Sy got between us and was taller than Barney but I didn't let go. Sy was facing me and I pulled this scumbag towards me as his chin pointed up and was squished against Sy's back and shoulder. I got another ten or twelve hard lefts straight down on him over Sy's shoulder before I was pulled off him.

Our medic boss needed medics, and if I had it to do over again I would, even though I know I was wrong. So after starting something he couldn't finish, I wound up spending the rest of the night down at central booking on Centre Street. But my boy's face was busted up good and I really didn't care about where I was.

So everyone who gets busted gets screened by an EMT before going into the bullpen. When the techs saw me they were shocked. When they found out whose ass I kicked, they came back with coffee and donuts for me, and gave me twelve dollars in quarters to make phone calls all night. When I got out, I was transferred to the Bronx and continued to act out. I quickly got myself in trouble over there then handed in my resignation.

My first job in EMS was an arrest and so was my last. In my own mind I went out on top. Either I was loved or hated, but everyone knew who I was. After I knocked out Barney, ninja medic cartoons appeared in every bathroom in every hospital. People graffittied "Free Dan Heidt" all over the station and someone even wrote you're my hero on my locker. People I had never met in my life were seeking me out to thank me, for my now legendary left.

I've been told I'm so pissed off because I know the way things should be. I learned that one man can not summon the future, but one man could change the present and that I needed to be a contender before I could be a champion. I learned from the best and I became the best. Together with my partners we made a difference. The guys I worked with over at 18 are the best fucking medics in the world, period. It was a privilege to work with them, and I sincerely thank all of you with my deepest respect. I'll be back to continue the whole fucking endless process… only just somewhere else.

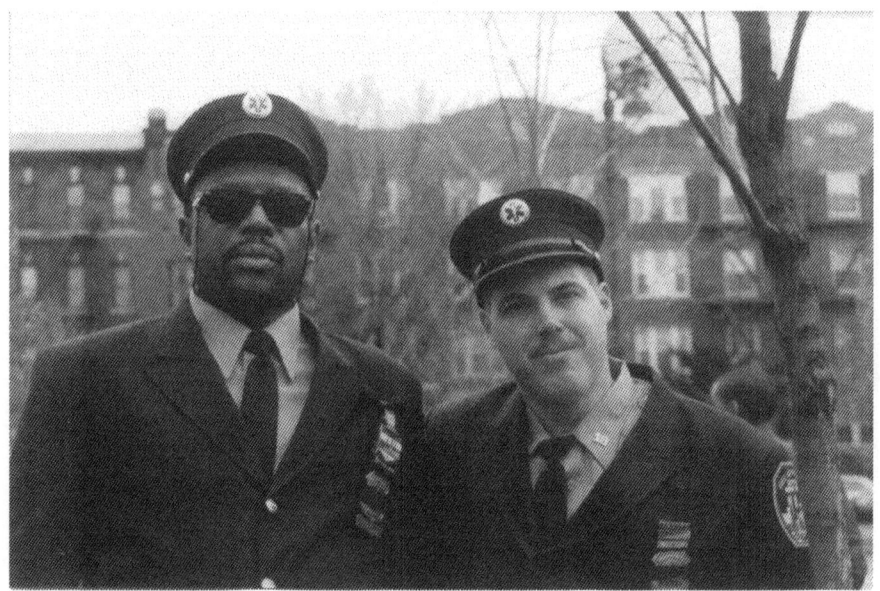

Me and Sy.

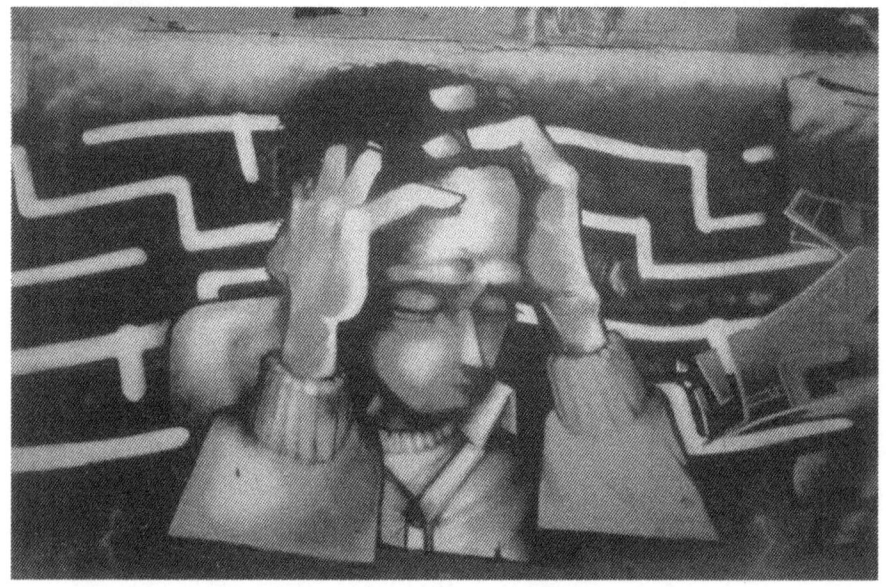

The way I feel at the end of the day.